Somatic Exercises

DISCLAIMER

The information provided in this book is intended for educational and informational purposes only. It is not a substitute for professional medical advice, diagnosis, or treatment. Always seek the advice of your physician or other qualified healthcare provider before starting any new fitness program or making any changes to an existing one. The author and publisher of this book are not responsible for any injury or health problems that may result from the use of the information in this book.

A Gift for You

Downloadable Somatic Yoga Exercise Chart

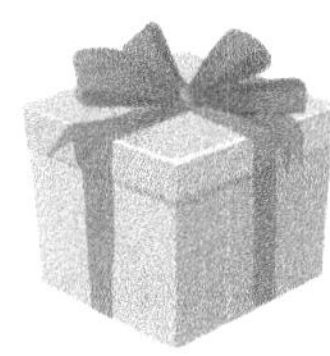

* A chart you can download.
  It helps you follow your exercises easily.

If you have any questions or simply want to thank us, please write to us at zealyonsfitness@gmail.com.

SCAN ME - - - - - ->

Contents

LYING EXERCISE

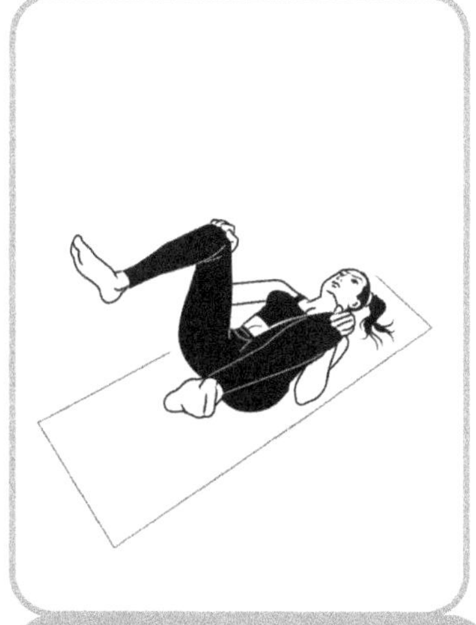

Hip Opening Circle

Page 09

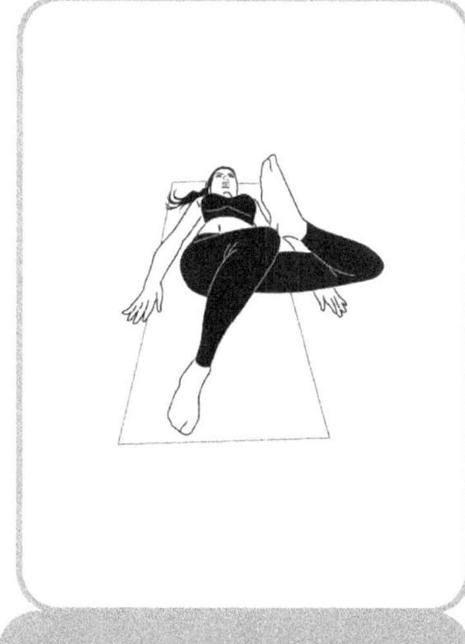

Hip Twist

Page 10

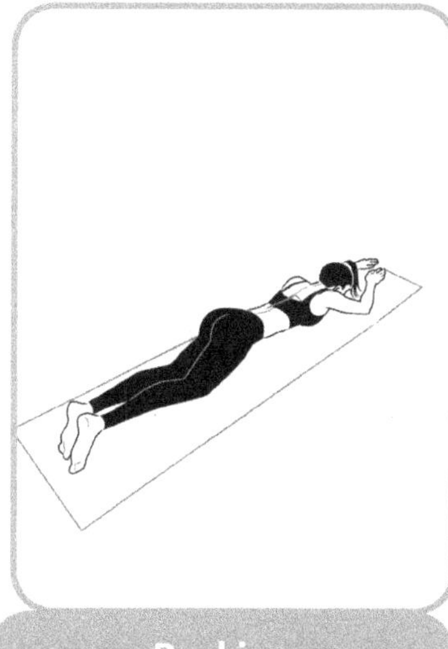

Rocking Hips

Page 11

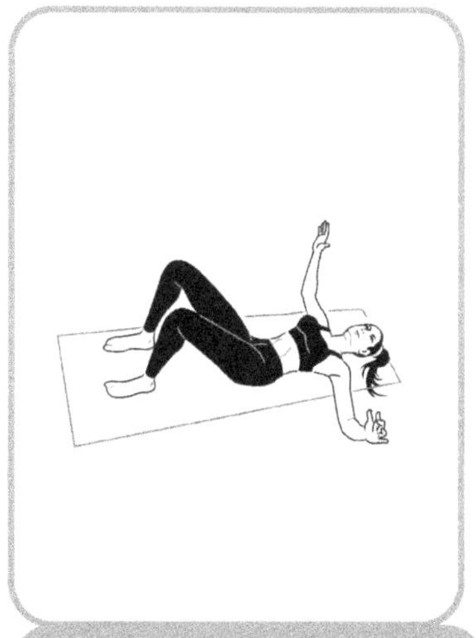

Lying Arm Windows

Page 12

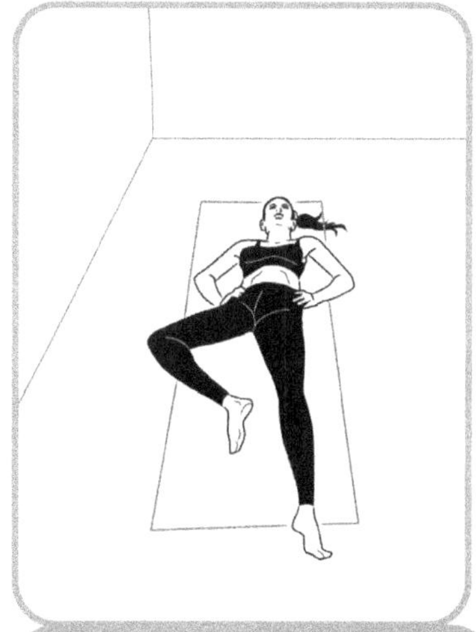

Releasing Bent Leg

Page 13

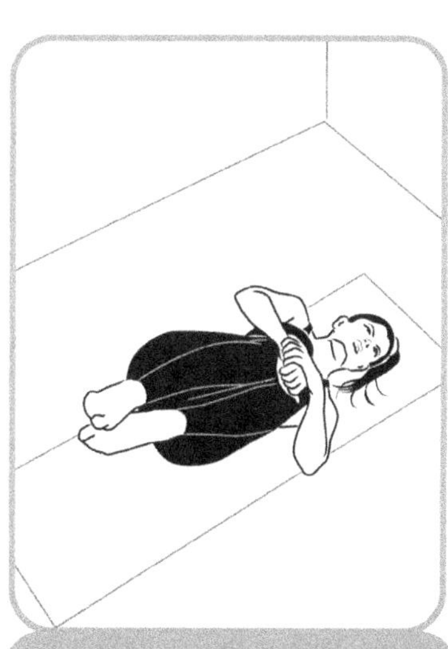

Swing Rock Pose

Page 14

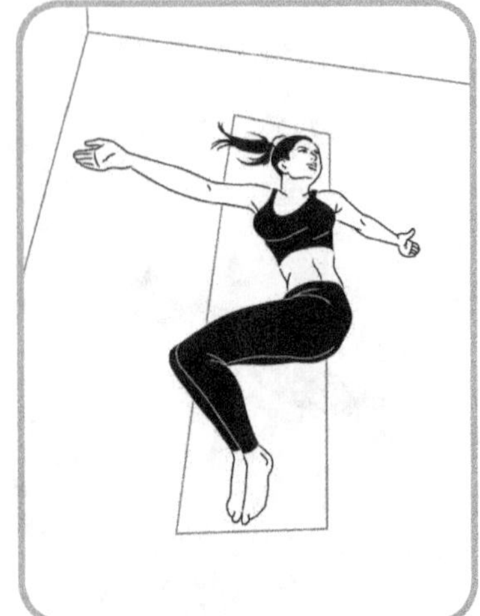

Side
Chest Opening

Page 15

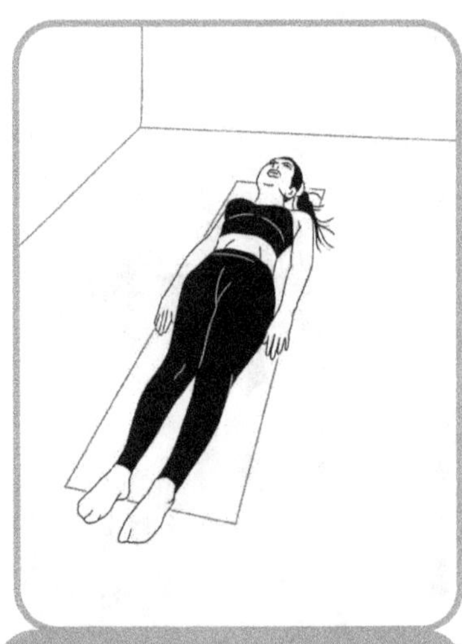

Whole Body Rocking

Page 16

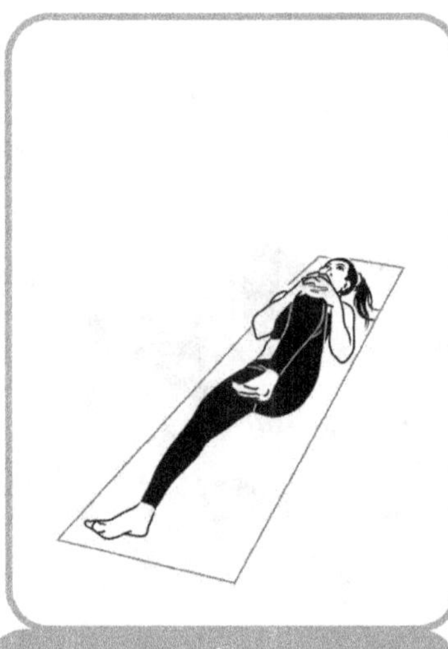

Lying
Knee Hugging

Page 17

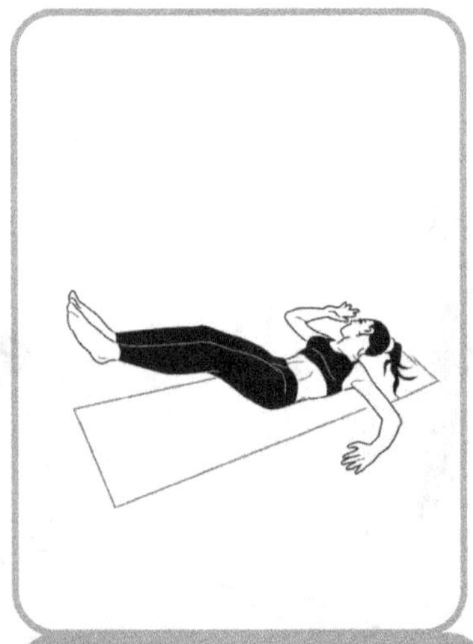

Alternating
Robot

Page 18

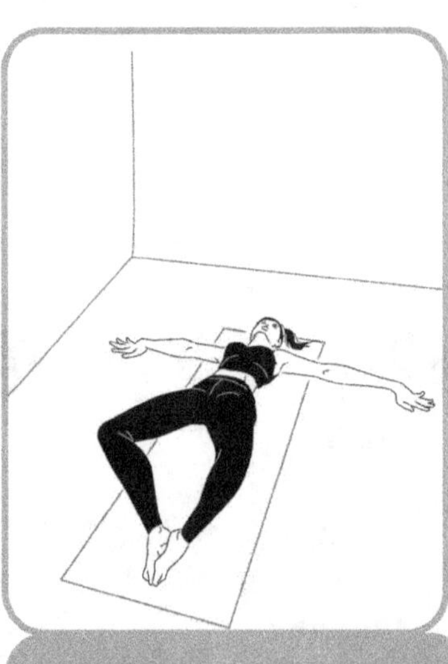

Hip
Lifting Star

Page 19

STANDING EXERCISES

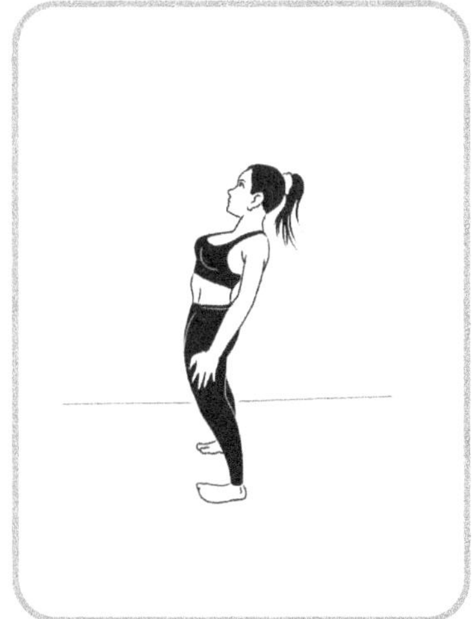

Spinal Swing

Page 20

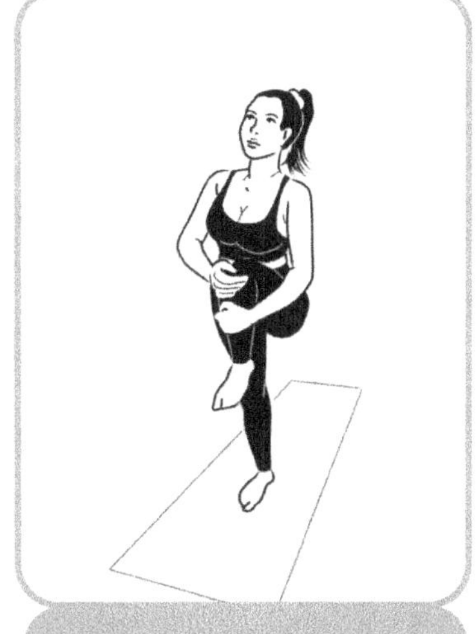

Knee Hugging

Page 21

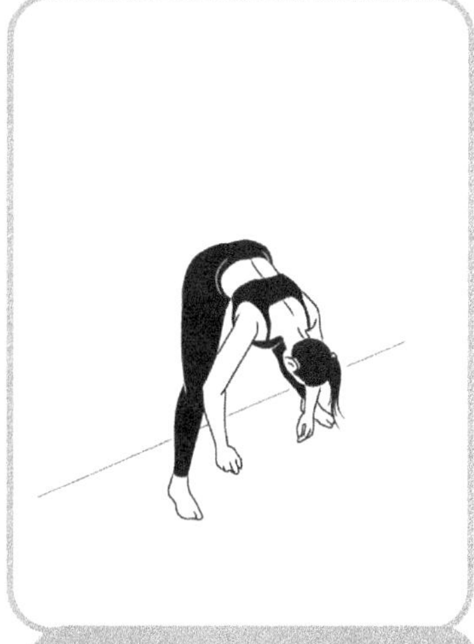

Circling Breath

Page 23

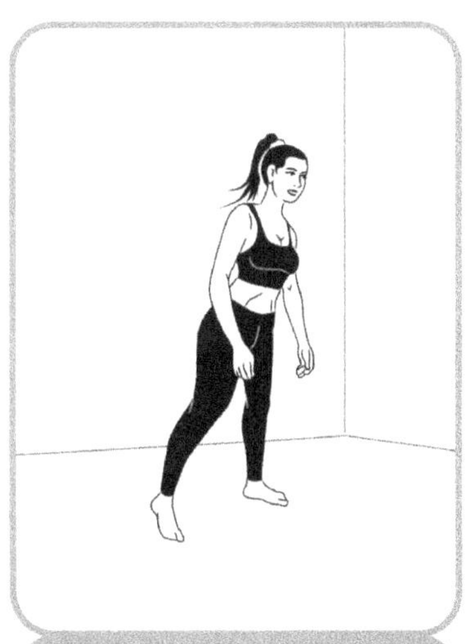

Sideways Flow

Page 24

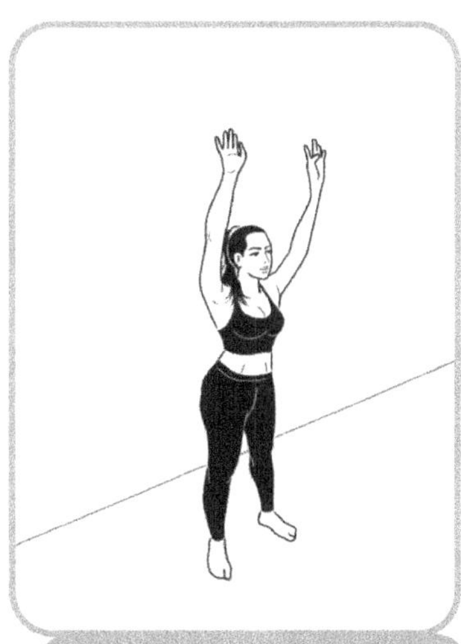

Sit & Raise

Page 25

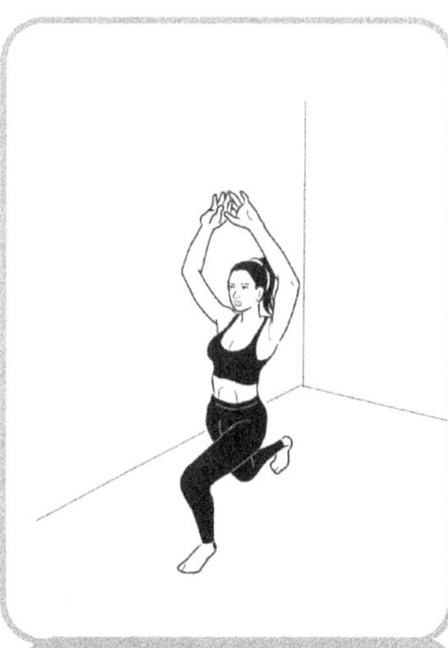

Releasing Lunge

Page 26

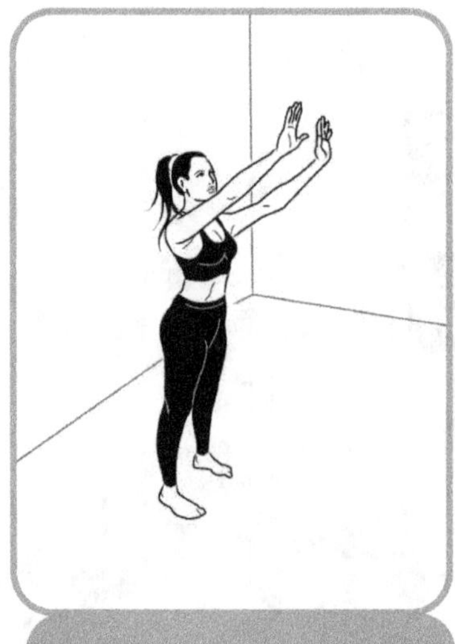

Energy Release

Page 27

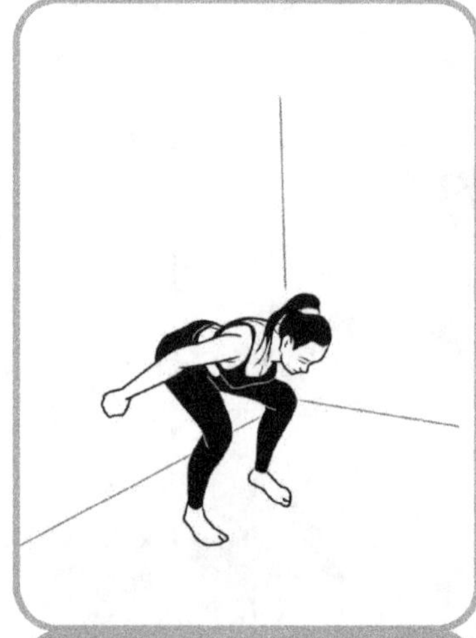

Stationary
Skiing

Page 28

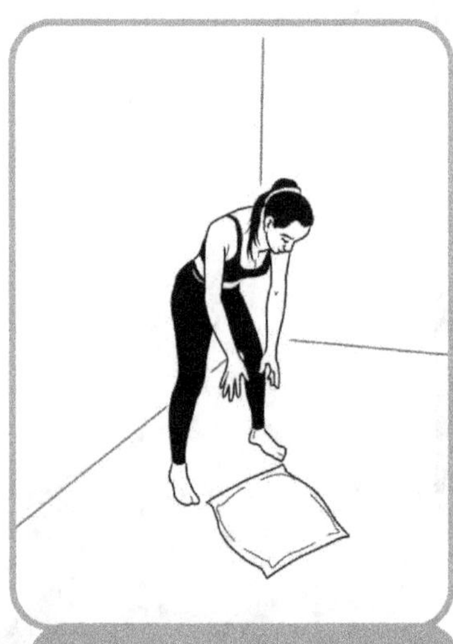

Pillow Slam

Page 29

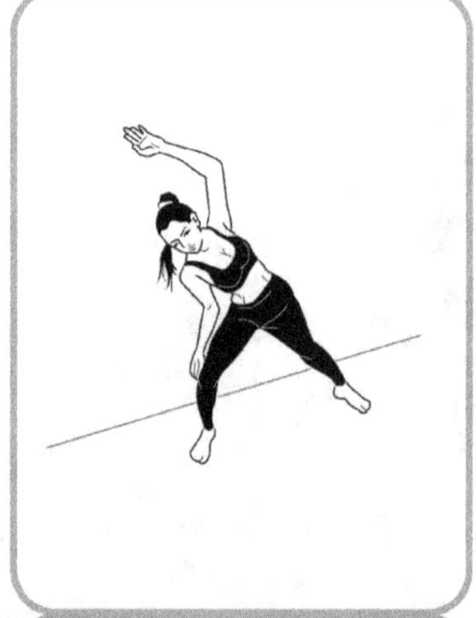

Side Lunge
And Extend

Page 30

SEATED & CRAWLING EXERCISES

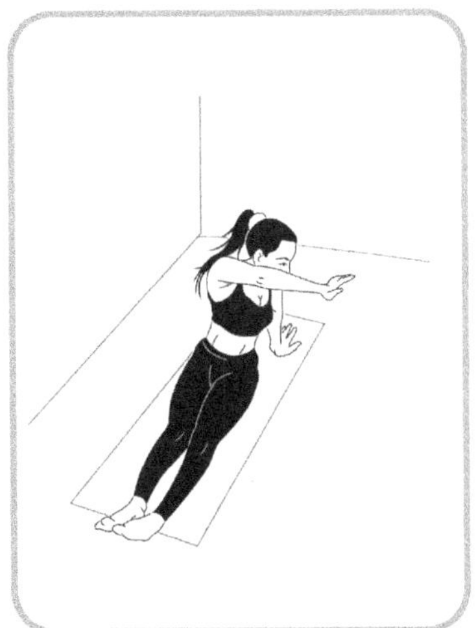

Trunk Reach Back

Page 31

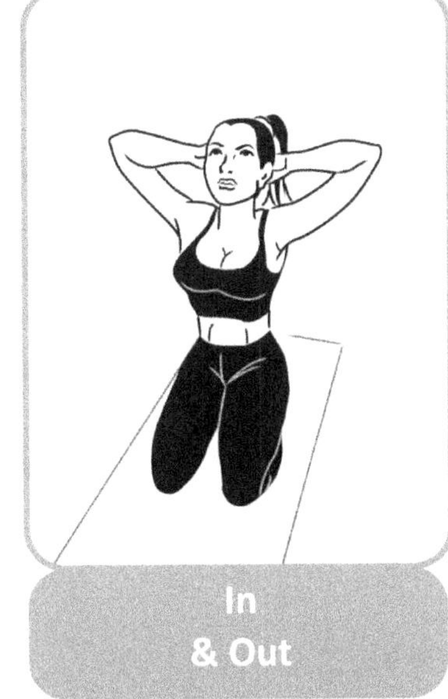

In & Out

Page 32

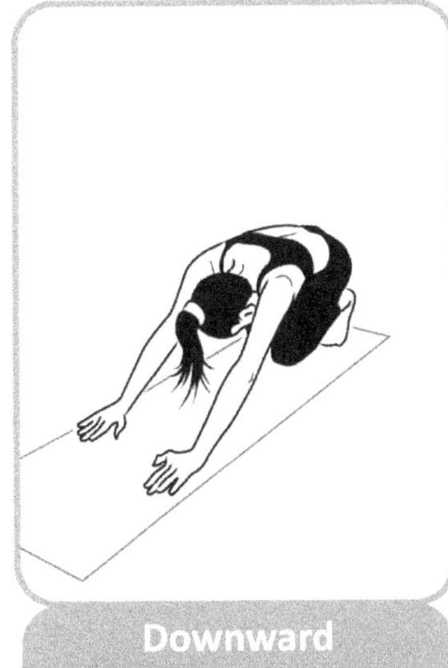

Downward Crawling

Page 33

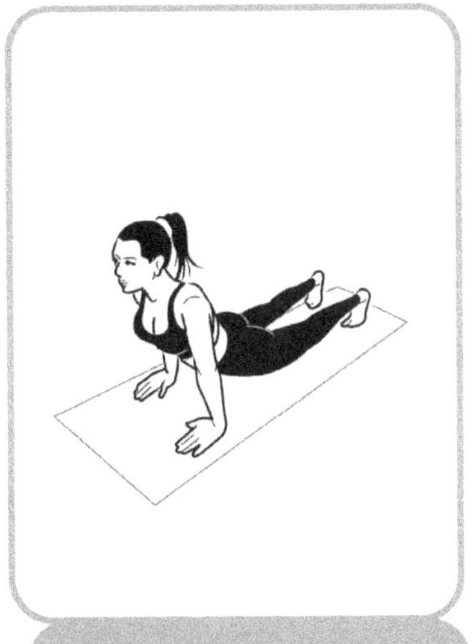

Downward Dog

Page 34

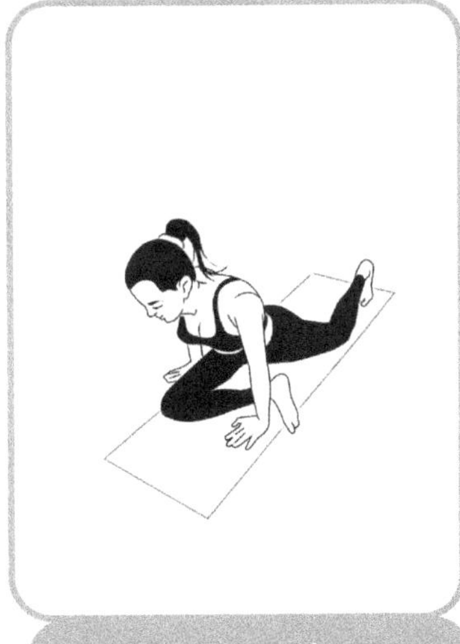

Dynamic Pigeon Pose

Page 35

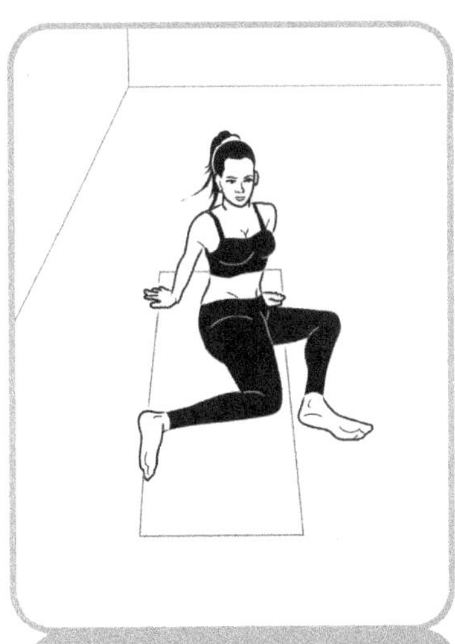

90/90s

Page 36

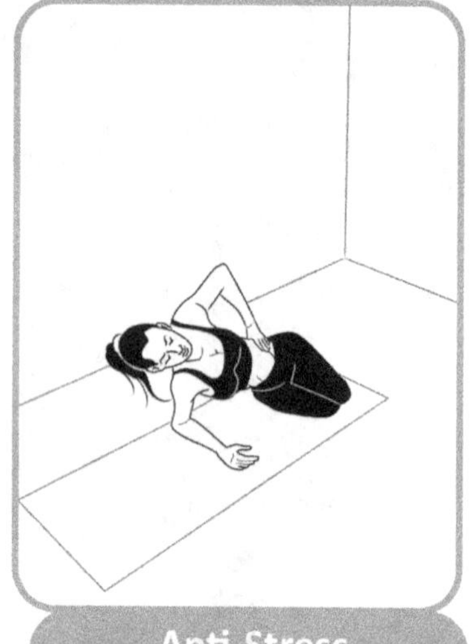

Anti-Stress Plank

Page 38

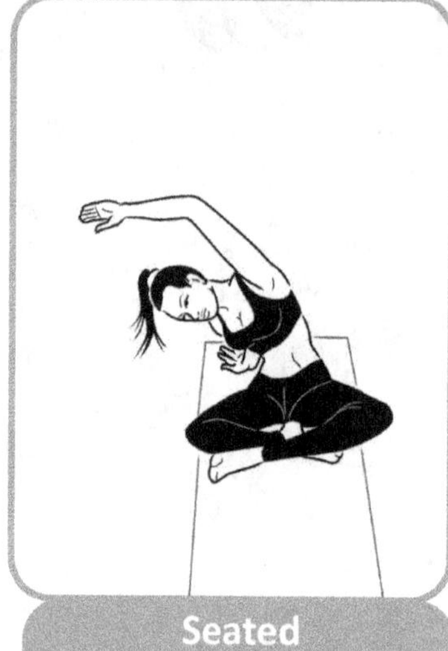

Seated Side Reach

Page 39

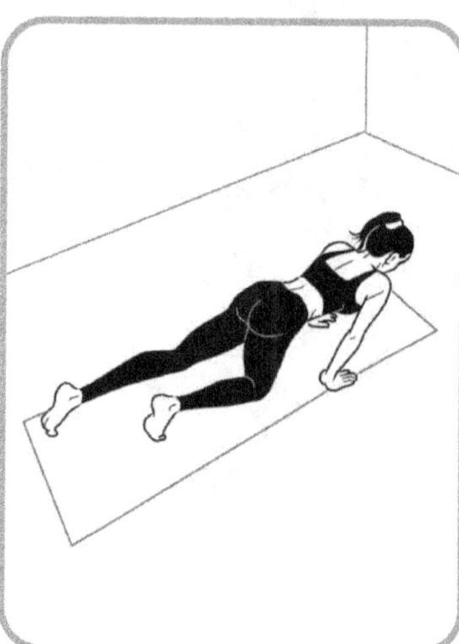

Top Point & Flex Pulses

Page 40

INTRODUCTION

I'm delighted that you've begun this journey, and I am confident that this book will be useful as a valuable resource for you as you seek to improve both your physical and mental health.

There are many advantages to somatic exercises, ranging from releasing trauma and improving flexibility to developing a stronger mind-body connection, releasing stress, feeling more in tune with your body, and regulating hormones. These activities address the interdependence of the body, mind, and spirit, going beyond simple physical exercise to represent a holistic approach to wellness. They can also contribute to weight loss and offer other benefits.

But without further ado, let's get started! Within this extensive manual, you will learn:

- A dedicated section addressing the most common questions about somatic exercises, covering topics such as their benefits, key information, tips, and how best to approach the exercises.

- Over 30 carefully selected exercises designed to make you feel better and happier than ever before. Each exercise is a step towards realizing your body's full potential and achieving a state of peace.

- A 28-day plan featuring an easy-to-follow exercise chart. This structured program ensures a daily progression, keeping you motivated and on track as you embark on your somatic journey.

- As a special bonus, we've included additional somatic daily practices that have the power to catapult your results to new heights.

And that's not all – expect much more insightful information, tips, and inspiration within these pages. Get ready to explore, learn, and experience the profound impact of Somatic Exercises on your life!

Also, for any question or doubt about the exercises and the training plan, feel free to email me at zealyonsfitness@gmail.com

Q&A

The most common questions answered

1. What are Somatic exercises?

Invented in the 1970s, somatics are practices aimed to improve healing from trauma, reduce stress, and enhance physical well-being through movements. These movements are characterized by a focus on the mind-body connection, and the practice is sensory, making the experience just as important as the movements themselves.

2. How long are the sessions?

The sessions can vary; they can range from 10 to 20 minutes long. It is highly suggested to be consistent with them, as only consistent training will bring you the benefits that you look for.

3. What are the benefits of this practice?

Somatic exercises offer numerous physical and mental and spiritual benefits. It is a complete practice, as other than improving flexibility and burning calories, it most importantly enhances the connection with your body and helps you release stress and anxiety. Moreover, it is also used to eliminate and heal from trauma.

4. Why choose this exercise method over other practices?

Due to its unique benefits and the fact that it mainly focuses on mental and spiritual well-being through movements, it is the perfect choice for anyone looking to feel better and less stressed while also improving their physical state.

5. What is the best way to read the book?

You will need to grasp the book's organizational structure, which consists of explanations of exercises followed by a comprehensive 28-day plan. Getting to know the exercises in advance enhances your comfort level when embarking on this 28-day program. The plan includes specific exercises to be performed. You can follow the exercise routine easier when you use the exercise chart. However a quick review of the exercises before starting each day is highly recommended.

6. How do I read the book with images and explanations?

It is suggested to have a look at the images first. By looking at them, you should be able to understand how to perform the exercise. Then, read the explanations that will guide you properly so that you'll perform the exercise perfectly.

7. Why is this good for weight loss even though you do not burn as many calories as other methods?

Somatic exercises are designed to alleviate stress and trauma, and effectively managing them is essential for overall well-being. When individuals experience improved mental and spiritual well-being, they are less prone to engaging in stress-induced behaviors like overeating and adopting a sedentary lifestyle. These mindful practices also contribute to weight loss. Furthermore, regular exercise not only burns calories but also enhances physical fitness. The positive impact on both mental and physical health encourages the adoption of healthier choices, creating a cycle of well-being. The plan incorporates exercises specifically aimed at reducing cortisol levels, the stress hormone, as elevated cortisol levels can impede weight loss.

8. What if I feel nausea during some exercises?

Ensure not to eat heavily before exercising. Adjust the intensity if it becomes too challenging. It is recommended to pause if you are not feeling okay and consult with a healthcare professional.

9. What should I do after the 28-day plan?

Once you finish the 28-day plan, you should feel quite familiar with the routine. My recommendation is to take 3 days completely off from training (long walks are fine), and then restart from day 15 until 28, increasing one set for each workout (so instead of repeating the sequence three or four times, you go up to four/five times). Definitely do not stop; the training and the process of self-improvement never stop.

10. If I do two workouts a day, would I feel and look better in half the time?

No, the training programs are studied carefully and designed for your best and quickest results. Doing more practices on the same day will not benefit you. It is important that you stay consistent and focused during the sessions for maximum results. For the best results, it is crucial that you do not think or do other things while performing the exercise; instead, focus on following the instructions.

11. Who can do somatic exercises?

Somatic exercises are aimed at those people who want to improve their mental health, release stress and trauma, as well as enhance their physical condition. Whether you want to lose weight, feel physically better, release stress, feel less tense and more present, or heal from trauma, this book is for you.

12. Are Somatic exercises useful for trauma healing?

Absolutely yes, various studies have been conducted on this. First of all, somatic exercises have been invented with this primary goal. In fact, trauma can be stored in the body through physical tension, and somatic exercises help you develop the mind-body connection as well as the relaxation of your body to slowly heal that trauma, also incorporating breathing techniques. Trauma can challenge the nervous system, and you'll notice how these exercises will massively relax you and make you feel more present if done correctly.

13. How do I know if I am releasing trauma?

It is a very subjective process, and it varies from person to person. Some individuals might experience sensations such as crying, laughing uncontrollably, feeling a sense of relief, or shaking. This can happen at different times during the plan. It might occur at the beginning of their journey (which is the minority), while others may start experiencing these sensations after weeks. Do not stress about it; it might happen that you will start to feel better, and slowly improve your trauma without feeling the need to cry or shake. Do not force these things to happen, as they will likely occur naturally and make you feel better.

14. Is there a best time of the day to do them?

There is no best time to do them as it is subjective. Some people experience better results doing these exercises in the evening at the end of the day, as it aims to release stress accumulated during the day and trauma, helping them go to sleep more relaxed. Other people prefer doing them in the morning as it sets them up for the rest of the day. I would suggest doing it in a time slot where you know you will not be disturbed; that is the most important thing. You can try different times of your day and see what feels best for you.

15. Is walking a somatic exercise?

Walking, when done mindfully, can be an effective component of somatic exercises. This is commonly known as "Walking Meditation," and the emphasis is on awareness of movement and foot contact with the ground. As a crucial part of somatic therapy, it promotes awareness and relaxation by establishing a connection of the body and mind. It is key that you do not use your phone while walking or listening to music. Multitasking would ruin the experience.

16. Is meditation a somatic exercise?

Certainly, meditation can be viewed as producing effects akin to somatic exercise. It strives to alleviate stress, encourages mindfulness, and, depending on the meditation technique, fosters a sense of connection with the body, establishing a mind-body relationship. Nevertheless, somatic practices prove more efficacious in releasing muscle tension and promoting an overall sense of improved well-being.

17. Do somatic exercises improve one's mood?

Somatic exercises do improve mood, and there are several reasons for this. Physical exercise improves mood; the combination of exercise and controlled breathing enhances presence. Moreover, it can help alleviate pain caused by poor posture or a low level of fitness, and it contributes to achieving better overall fitness. On top of this, when engaging in physical exercise, the human body releases dopamine, a neurotransmitter that regulates mood. Its release is linked to improved mood and increased happiness.

18. What to focus on during the exercises?

When doing somatic exercises, the main thing that sets them apart is their focus on feeling and sensation. It's crucial to pay attention to your breath and how your body feels. Don't try to do multiple things at once. Your mind might wander, but just let those thoughts go and go back to focusing on your breath and body sensations. This is key for a successful practice.

19. What does the mind-body connection mean?

Developing a mind-body connection is a slow process. We are often too focused on tasks, external matters, and even people who work out daily tend to neglect how their body is actually feeling. Developing a mind-body connection helps in understanding which areas of the body are tense, as it will assist you in comprehending where you hold trauma. This is crucial because it makes you aware of the tensions in your body, enabling you to relieve them through exercises. Once you establish a strong mind-body connection, you will feel more in control of your body, more connected to it, and better able to improve your physical and mental health quickly.

20. What positive changes can I expect in myself after finishing the whole book?

Following the plan methodically will help you:

- Reduced stress and improved mindfulness.

- Enhanced happiness, weight loss, improved fitness and more flexibility.

- Healing from trauma.

- Better understanding of your body.

- Stronger mind-body connection.

If you have any questions or doubts, feel free to contact me at zealyonsfitness@gmail.com, and I'll be happy to assist you the best I can about somatic exercises and workouts!

ENJOY YOUR BONUS HERE

7 Daily Practices, other than the daily exercises, I genuinely recommend (at least one of them a day) to feel better and enhance the results you'll have with these workouts!

Experiencing difficulties with your bonus download? Feel free to reach out to us at zealyonsfitness@gmail.com , and our team or I will promptly assist you!

LYING EXERCISE

HIP OPENING CIRCLE

Great way to gently release stiffness on your hips and rebalance your cortisol levels.

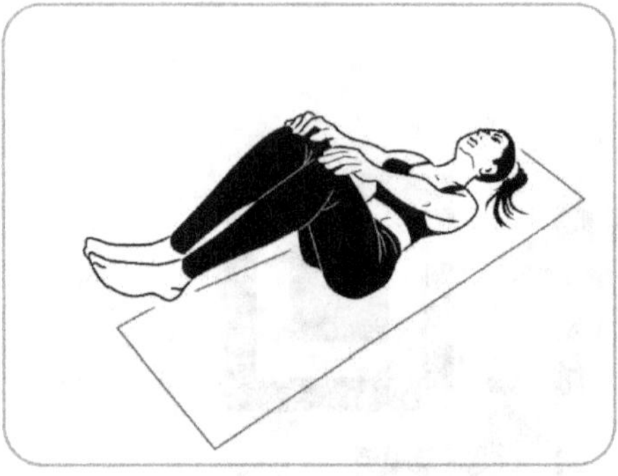

- Start by lying down on the mat with your knees bent, feet up, and hands on your knees. Breathe gently.

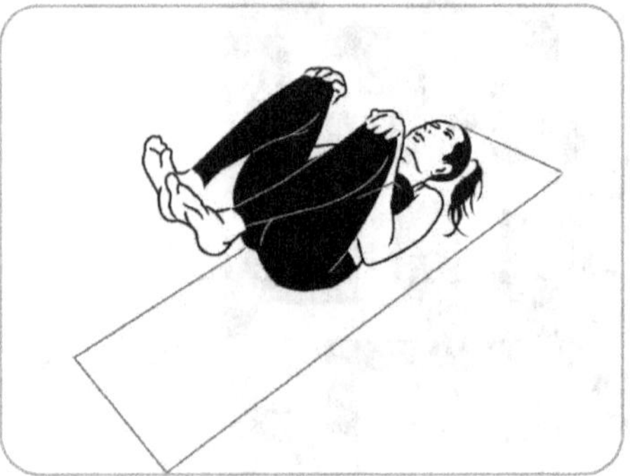

- From there, bring your knees towards your chest keeping your knees close to each other.

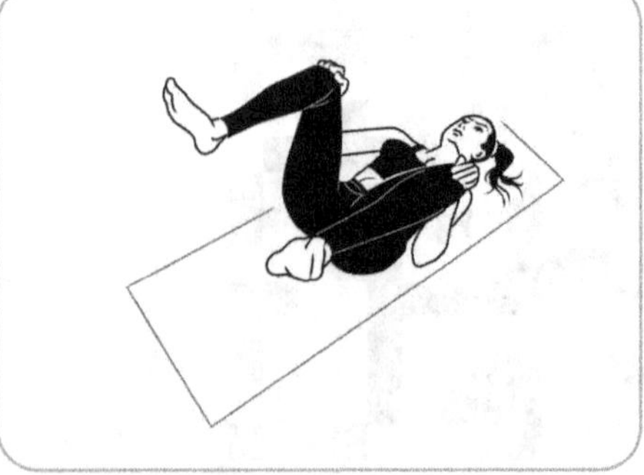

- Then, open up your knees as shown and slowly, come back into starting position, as if you were to draw a circle with your knees.

- Repeat for the mentioned reps.

Extra Tips:

When you perform the exercise the first time, you may experience nausea as your muscles release years / decades of tension. Drink plenty of water before and after the workout to prevent nausea.

Also, as you bring the knees to your chest it is quite common to hold your breath - This is a common mistake that should be avoided. Try exhaling fully and release into the position.

HIP TWIST

Great exercise for increasing lower body mobility and back flexibility. Breathe out all the tension while performing the exercise.

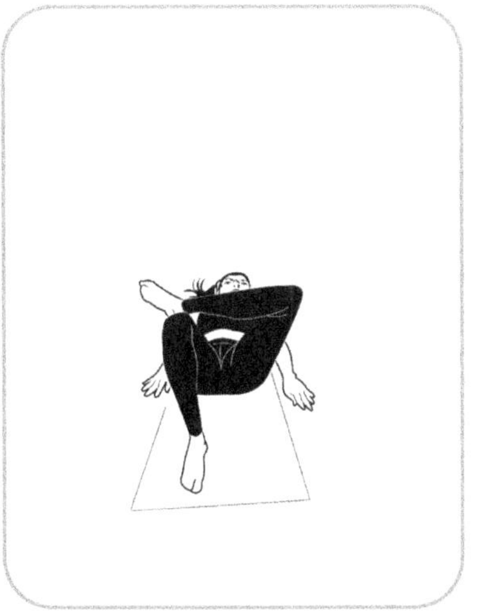

- Assume a prone position. Bend your right leg with your right foot fully on the ground. Then, bend your left leg so that the outside of your left ankle touches your right knee - your left glute should feel slightly stretched. Keep your arms on the ground.

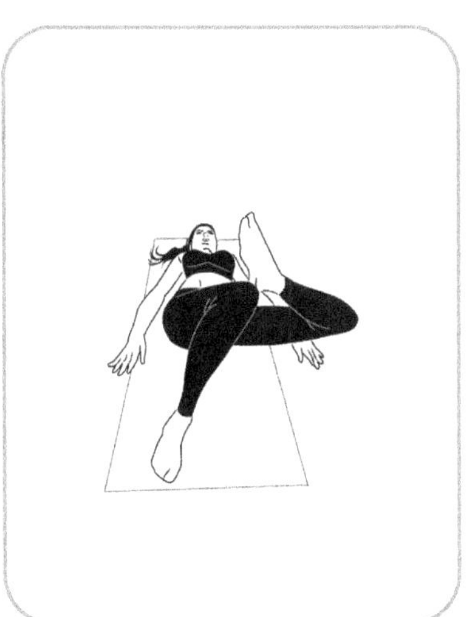

- Keep your back to the floor as you rotate your hips to the left with your left knee getting closer to the floor. Hold the position for 1 second.

- Come back to the starting position, and repeat the movement for the mentioned reps . Lastly, repeat it on the other side.

Extra Tips:

Remind yourself to pay attention to your breathing, exhaling as you rotate your hips outwards, and gently inhale as you come back to the starting position.

If you have any questions or doubts, feel free to contact me at

zealyonsfitness@gmail.com**, and I'll be happy to assist you the best I can about**

somatic exercises and workouts!

ROCKING HIPS

Great exercise to release the toxins produced within your body from unprocessed emotions.

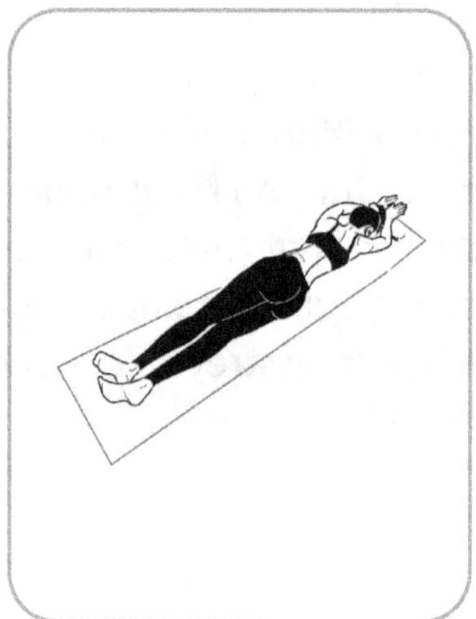

- Lying down with your belly on the floor, feet together and arms over your head.
- From there, move your hips towards one side.

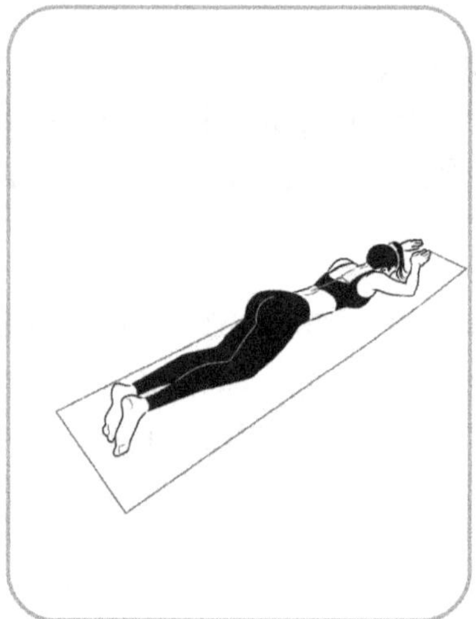

- Then, move them smoothly towards the other side.
- Keep repeating the sequence from side to side for the mentioned times.

LYING ARM WINDOWS

Great exercise to get rid of anxiety spikes.

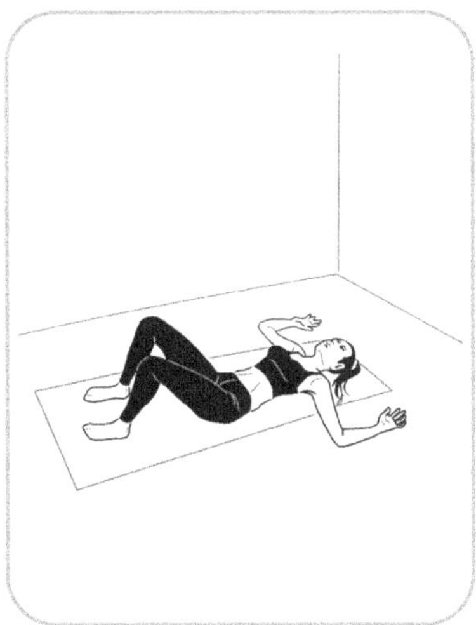

- Start lying down on your back with your knees bent and feet on the floor. Arms at 90° angle with forearms on the floor.

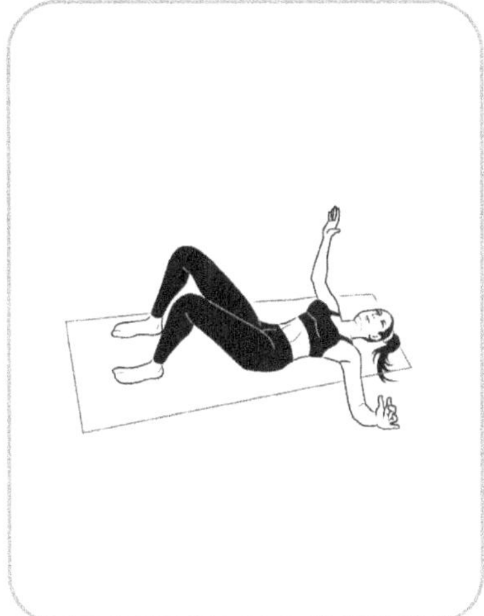

- Then, while exhaling gently, lift your forearms vertical to the floor. Hold it for 1 second.

- Finally, come back into the starting position whilst inhaling through your nose. Repeat the movement for the mentioned reps.

Extra Tips:

The focus here is to perform the movement gently to mobilize the upper back/ shoulder area that often stores lots of unprocessed emotions and trauma.

RELEASING BENT LEG

Fantastic movement to reduce excess levels of cortisol, helping balancing hormonal levels.

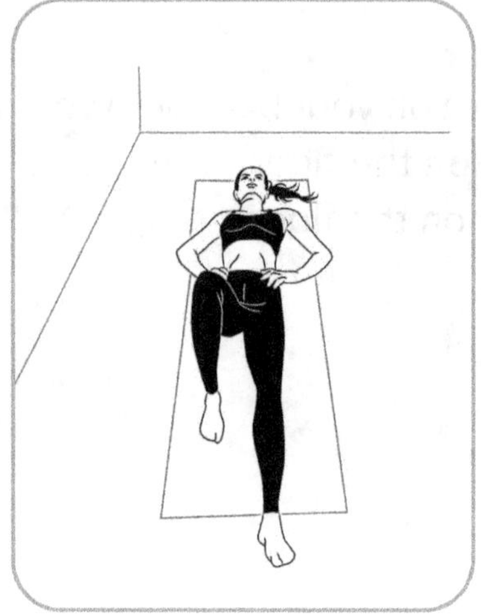

- Lay down with your back on the mat, your hands on your waist and your left leg straight. Right leg bent as shown.

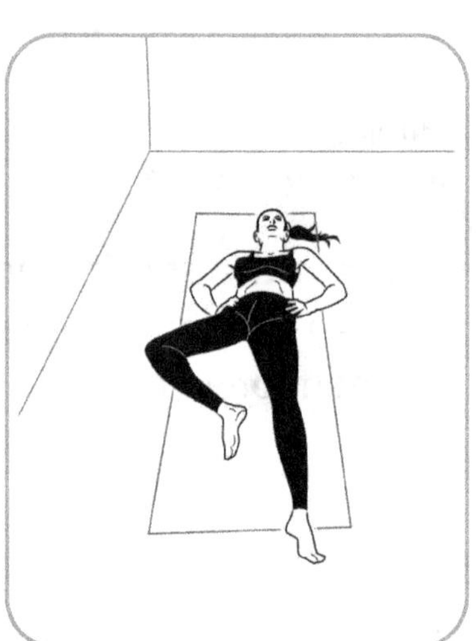

- From there, gently move it towards the floor. Exhale through your mouth as you do so. Hold it for 1 second.

- Then, come back into the starting position as you inhale.

- Repeat the sequence for the mentioned reps. Lastly, repeat it on the other side - having your right leg straight on the floor, and your left leg bent.

Extra Tips:

As you exhale while opening up your leg, focus on relaxing the muscles around the hips. It will make the exercise more effective.

SWING ROCK POSE

It improves balance, flexibility, and relieves lower back pain, as well as reducing tension in your hips and lower back area.

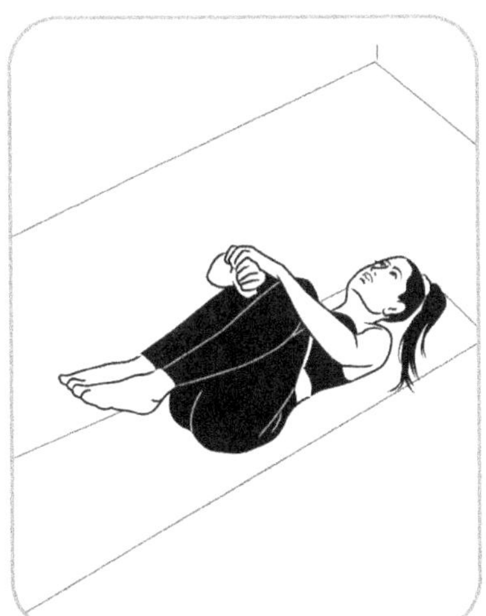

- Lie on your back and bring your knees to your chest. Exhale gently.

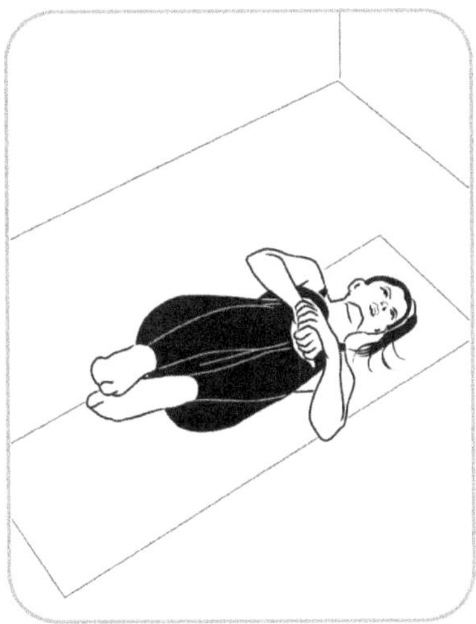

- Then, move your body in a gentle rocking motion from side to side, from left to right. Ensure that your spine remains on the mat throughout. For best results, move slowly and with gentleness.

- Perform the sequence for the mentioned seconds.

Extra Tips:

This is a great exercise to get comfortable in a position you probably haven't been in for decades. Don't worry; focus on gentle breathing, relaxing all the muscles as you do so, and moving gently from side to side. In a few seconds, you'll feel calmer and more serene.

SIDE CHEST OPENING

Exercise to improve chest and shoulder flexibility. Breathe deeply to relieve tension. It improves posture and body alignment.

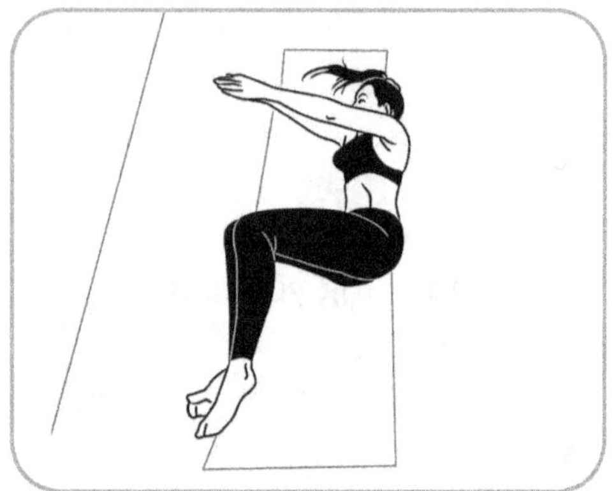

- Lie on your right side on the floor in a fetal position to begin. Also, extend your arms on the floor in front of you.

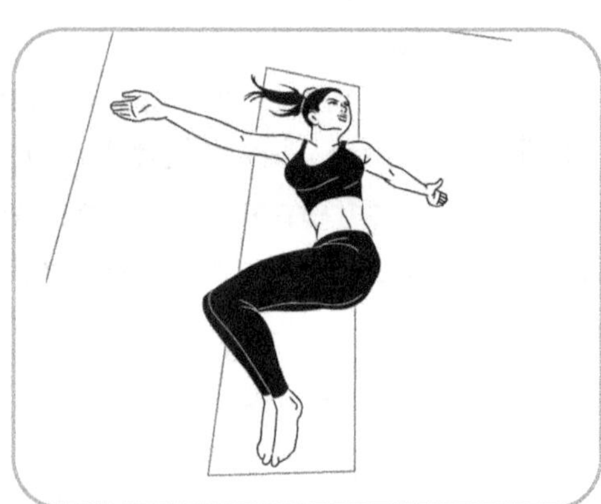

- Next, visualize using your left hand to draw a semicircle in the air. While keeping your right hand on the ground, open your chest, and place your left hand on the floor on the other side. You're going to 'open up' your chest with this action. Hold this posture for one full breath—both inhale and exhale.

- Then, come back to the starting position, and repeat for the mentioned reps.

- Finally, repeat it on the other side by lying on your left side.

Extra Tips:

At first, you might have some difficulty extending your arm completely on the floor as you open up your chest. No worries; this is quite normal. Make sure to exhale deeply as you get into that position and relax your chest/shoulder area. By the second week, you should already notice improvements!

WHOLE BODY ROCKING

Connecting the body from toe to head. It promotes body awareness and relaxation.

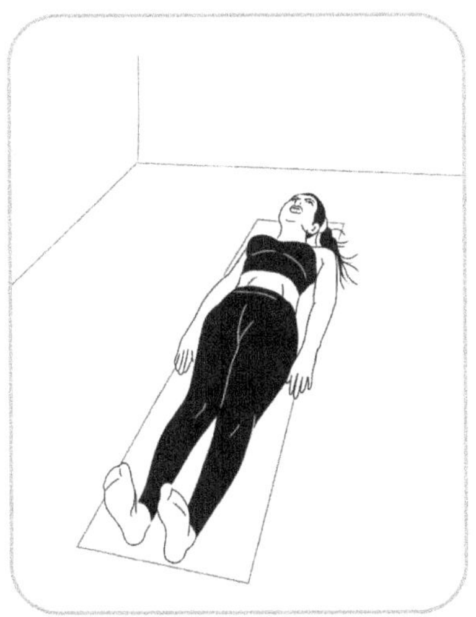

- Lie on your back, legs straight and arms next to your body.

- Lift your toes and inhale through your nose, as shown in the first image. Hold the position, inhaling for 3 to 5 seconds to feel the energy flow through your body.

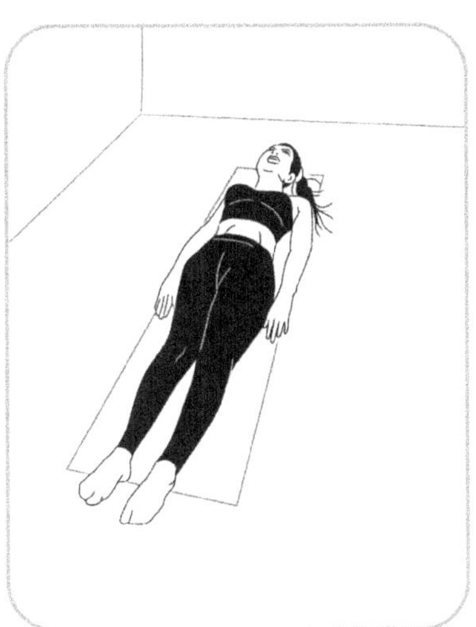

- Then, extend your toes away from you and exhale gently through your mouth. Hold the position for 5 to 8 seconds, allowing your body to release muscle tension.

- Repeat the sequence for the given number of seconds.

Extra Tips:

You'll know you're doing it right if, during the exercise, you feel your body rocking up and down. It might take a bit, but eventually, you'll get there.

LYING KNEE HUGGING

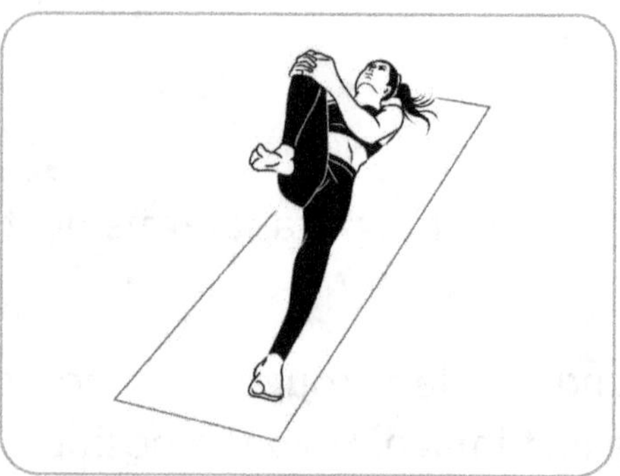

- Lie on your back with your left leg extended and hug your right knee at chest level. Relax your shoulders and neck while on the mat. Hold the position for 3 seconds while exhaling fully.

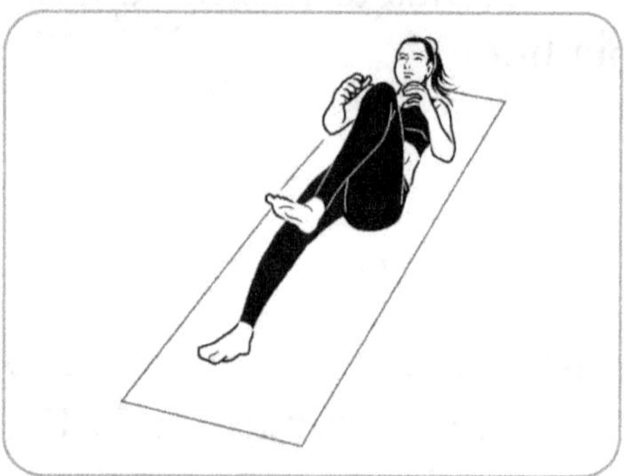

- Switch legs. Bring the right leg down first, then lift the left one up. Perform the movement slowly.

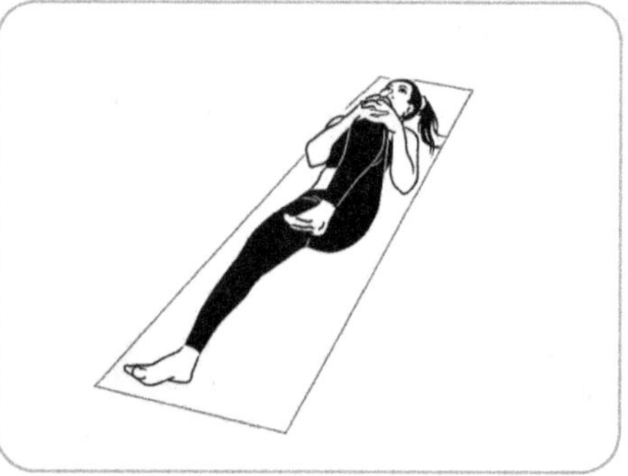

- Repeat on the other side, holding the position for 3 seconds and exhaling fully.

- Perform the movement for the specified number of times, alternating sides.

Extra Tips:

For the best results, move slowly. Remember to exhale through your mouth. This is a great exercise for increasing flexibility. Do not worry if it is difficult to bring the knee close to the chest while keeping your back on the mat. Maintain your back flat on the mat and your knee as close to your chest as possible. You will improve as you practice.

ALTERNATING ROBOT

Fantastic movement to release trauma and tension in your shoulders and neck, as well as improving posture and strengthening your core area.

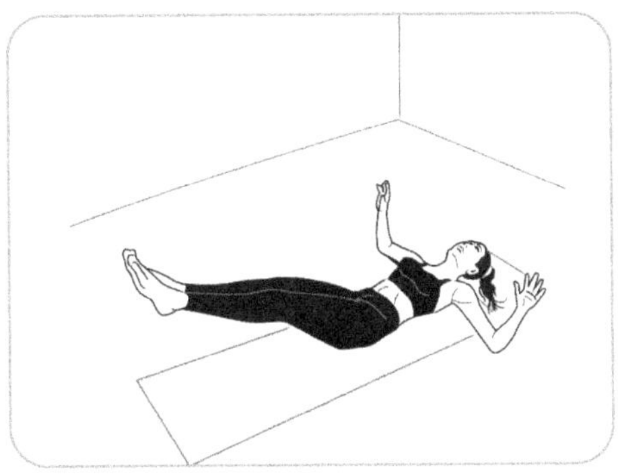

- Start by lying on the floor with your back on it and lift your legs as shown. Keep your arms open to the side with your forearms lifted - this is the starting position.

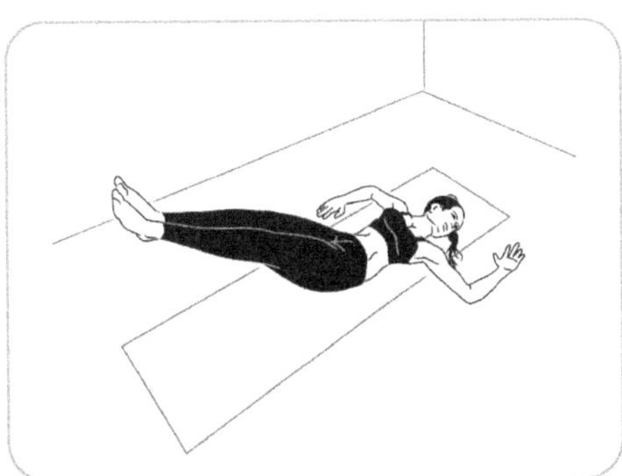

- Then, move your left forearm to the floor with your left hand pointing over your head, whilst the right forearm goes to the floor with your hand pointing down towards the feet - As you do so rotate your head towards the left hand.

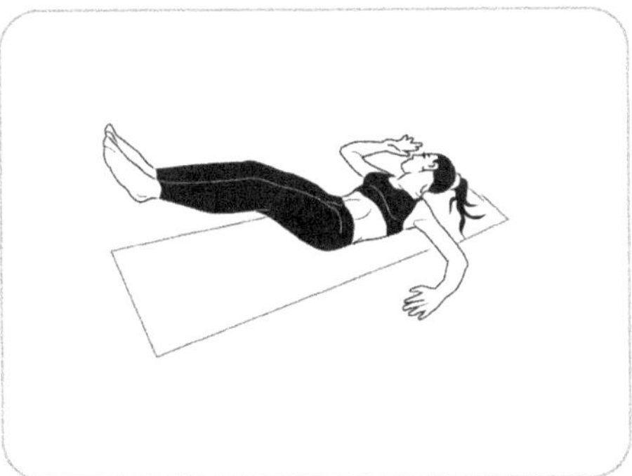

- Then, come back to the starting position, and repeat on the other side.
- Perform the mentioned reps alternating the sides, as shown.

Extra Tips:

It will engage your core as well as improve your posture in ways not many exercises do. If this is too difficult, put your legs on the floor, and when you feel comfortable, perform the exercises as shown in the images.

HIP LIFTING STAR

Exercise to strengthen and release tension from your glutes and groins.

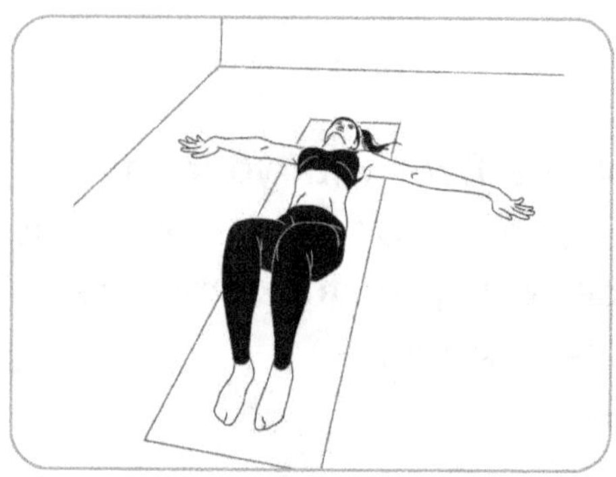

- Lie on your back with legs bent and feet flat on the ground, close to each other. Fully extend your arms to the side, forming a 90-degree angle with your trunk.

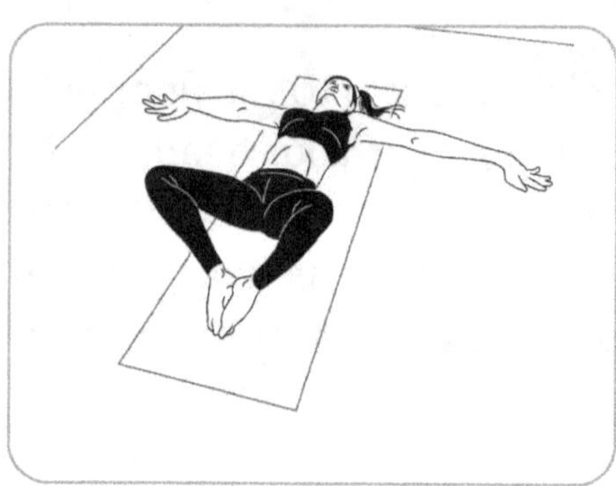

- Inhale and let your knees drop sideways, bringing your soles together, as shown. Feel the stretch in your groin as you do this. (You may also notice an arch in your lower back; this is normal.) Maintain that position for 2 seconds while breathing gently.

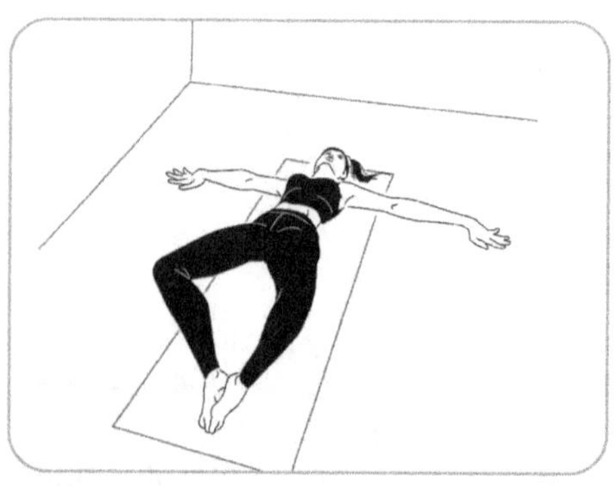

- Next, lift your hips while keeping your soles together, knees open, and arms in the same position.

- Exhale completely and slowly bring your buttocks to the mat, returning your knees to their starting position. Do it slowly and deliberately.

- You have completed your first repetition. Repeat for the specified number of repetitions.

STANDING EXERCISES

SPINAL SWING

Spinal mobility exercises improve flexibility and reduce pain as well as strengthening your mind-body connection.

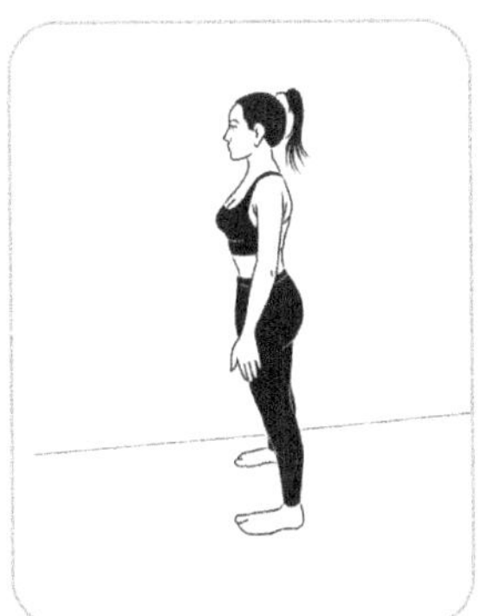

- Begin in a standing position with your arms by your sides and your entire body in a straight line.

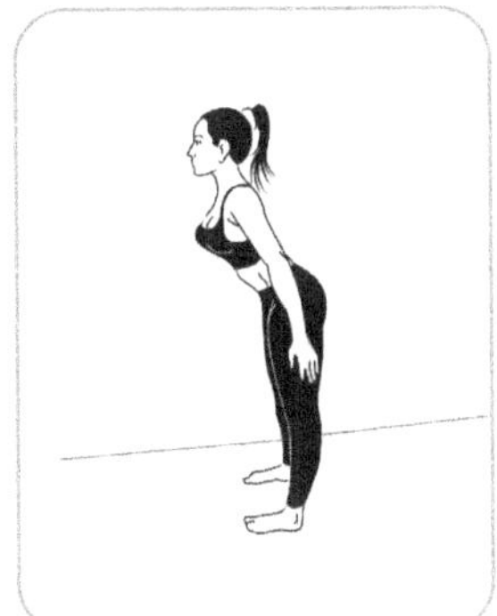

- Then, gently and smoothly bring your chest and head forward by moving your spine.

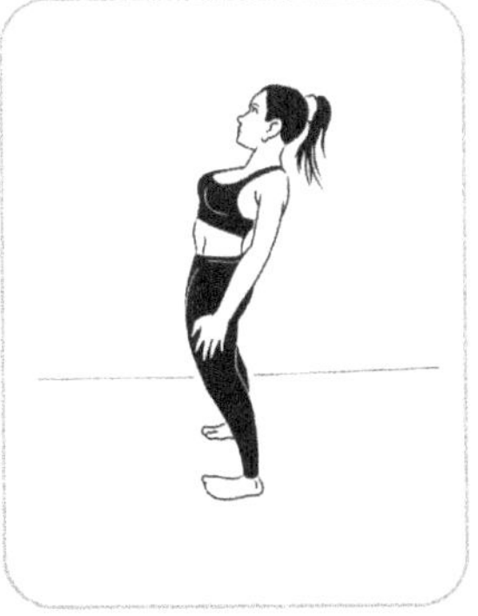

- Next, return to the starting position while pushing your belly forward.
- Continue this sequence for the mentioned time.

Extra Tips:

Let's keep it easy: Maintain a straight posture and alternately bring your belly and chest forward while moving your spine like a wave. Additionally, the slower and more mindful you perform the movement, the better you'll feel afterward.

KNEE HUGGING

Great exercise to improve balance and coordination, as well as lower body mobility. "Hugging" promotes positive emotions.

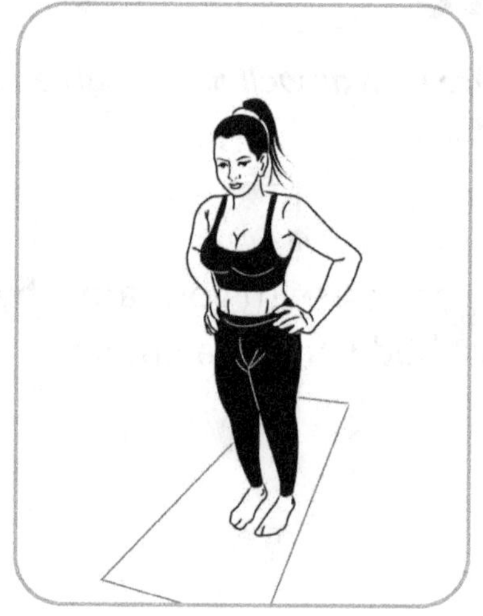

- Begin by standing on the mat with hands on the side. Inhale gently.

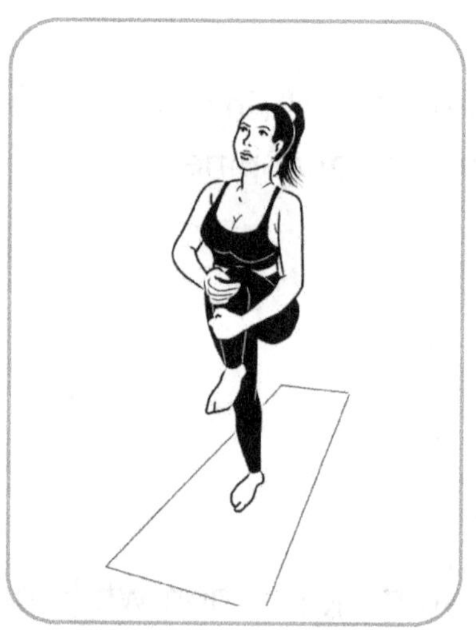

- Then, using both hands, bring one knee close to your chest while keeping only one foot on the floor. Concentrate on deep, controlled breathing, inhaling through the nose and exhaling through the mouth.

- Maintain the position for 10 seconds, breathing gently throughout.

- Then, come back to the starting position, and repeat on the other leg. Repeat for the mentioned reps, alternating sides.

Extra Tips:

If you lack balance, try focusing on a specific point on the floor a few feet away from you. 'Fixing' your gaze on something typically makes you feel more balanced.

Additionally, if 10 seconds is too long, try holding each position for 5 seconds. Over time, your balance will improve, and you will be able to hold the position for 10 seconds without difficulty.

If you have any questions or doubts, feel free to contact me at <u>zealyonsfitness@gmail.com,</u> and I'll be happy to assist you the best I can about somatic exercises and workouts!

CIRCLING BREATH

Great exercise for releasing stress and improving balance. Perfect for connecting with your body.

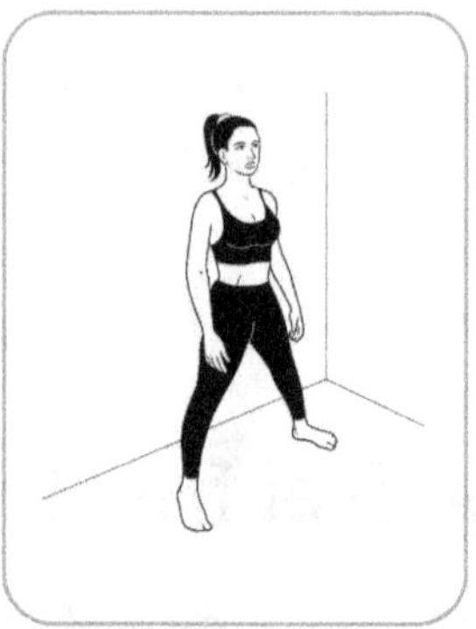

- Stand with your legs spread and your arms to the sides.

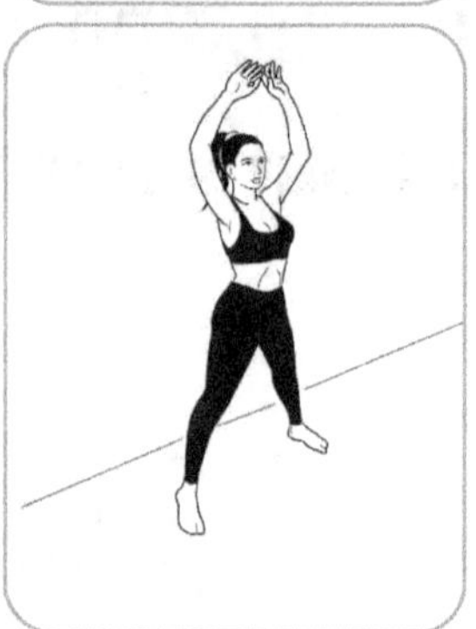

- Bring your arms over your head, and inhale through your nose, fully inflating your chest. Imagine absorbing all the positive energy around you. This step should only take one to two seconds.

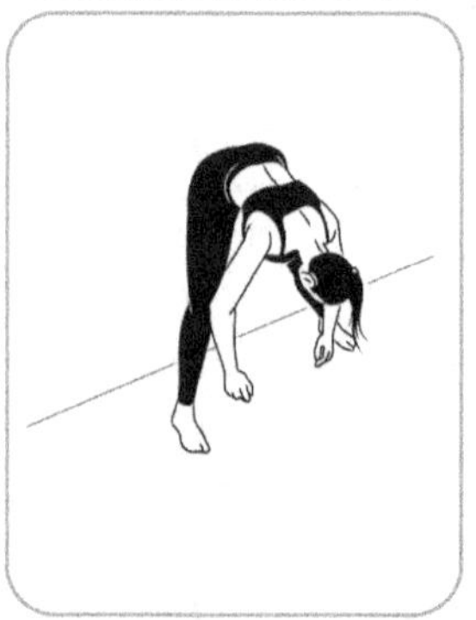

- Then, lower your trunk and arms to the floor while exhaling fully and releasing all of your emotions. This step should take two to three seconds.
- Then, return to the starting position and repeat for the specified number of repetitions.

Extra Tips:

Great exercise for reconnecting with your body and finding relief in a few deep breaths. The more you can spread your legs, the better, especially as you exhale and relax your back.

SIDEWAYS FLOW

This exercise aims at enhancing the connection between body and mind as you have to constantly switch your balance side to side.

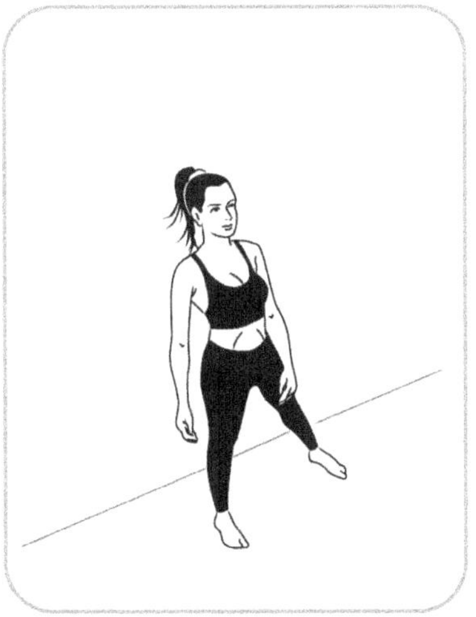

- Begin by standing with your feet slightly wider than hip width apart and your arms by your sides.

- Then, as shown in the image, step slightly to the side with your right foot and balance on it. Hold that position for 1 second, focusing on how your body feels as you maintain this

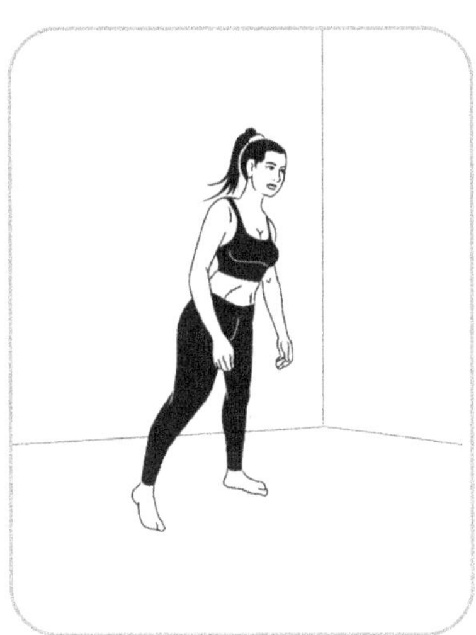

- Next, repeat the movement on the left side, balancing on your left foot.

- Keep alternating between these two movements for the mentioned seconds.

Extra Tips:

It is critical that you pay close attention to your body while performing this exercise. Concentrate on your feet for improved balance. Continue to breathe normally, without interference. While some people find it natural to hold their breath, avoid doing so for maximum effectiveness.

SIT & RAISE

Weight loss exercise combining lower body and cardio exercises. It also enhances coordination.

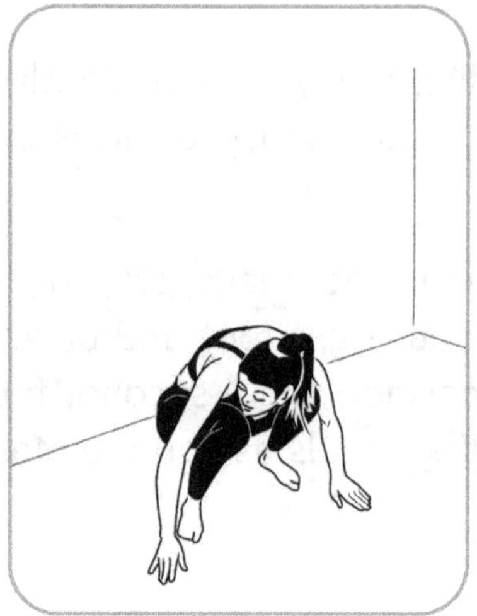

- Begin in a deep squat position with arms alongside the body, inhaling through your nose.

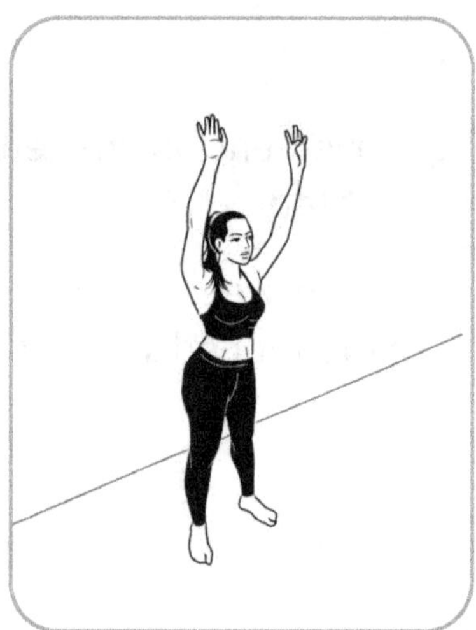

- Next, stand up with your arms extended overhead, mimicking the blooming of a flower. Exhale fully, imagining releasing all the accumulated tension.

- Then, return to the starting position and repeat for the mentioned reps.

Extra Tips:

This one is quite challenging cardiovascularly. Ideally, do it non-stop. There is no need to perform it fast; a nice and steady movement for the specified number of seconds works amazingly.

RELEASING LUNGE

Great exercise for lower body strength, mind-body connection and coordination.

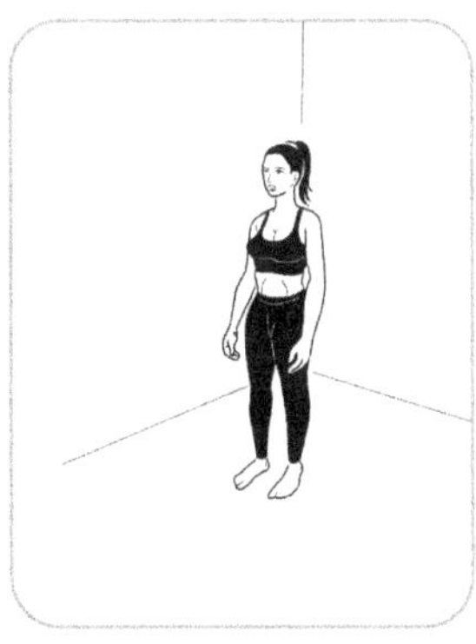

- Stand hip-width apart with arms at your sides. Inhale through your nose, paying attention to how your body feels.

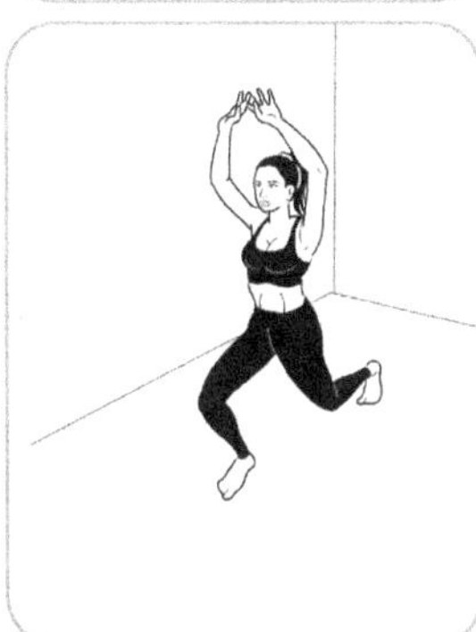

- Then, lunge forward with your right leg (aim for your right thigh to be parallel to the floor, and your left knee nearly touching the ground). As you extend your arms, exhale fully.

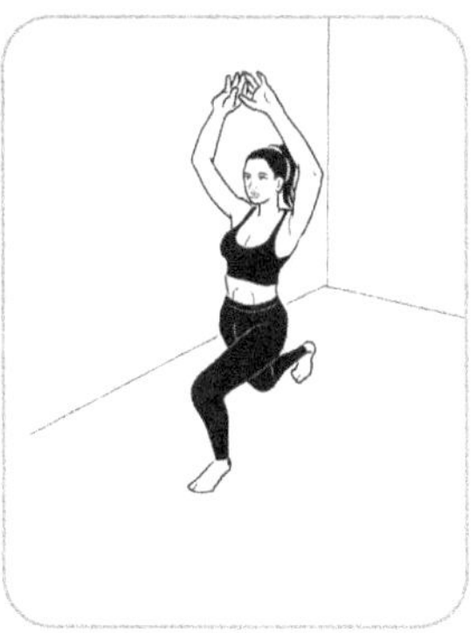

- Next, return to the starting position and repeat on the left side, as shown. Keep alternating sides for the specified number of repetitions.

Extra Tips:

If you lack balance, I recommend looking at a specific point a few feet away. This will help you keep your body stable. Also, inhale as you return to the starting position. Concentrate on releasing all tension as you lunge and inhaling all the energy around you as you return to your starting position.

ENERGY RELEASE

Perfect exercise to release stress and tension. Proper breathing, as it will be mentioned, plays a key role in maximizing the benefits of the exercise.

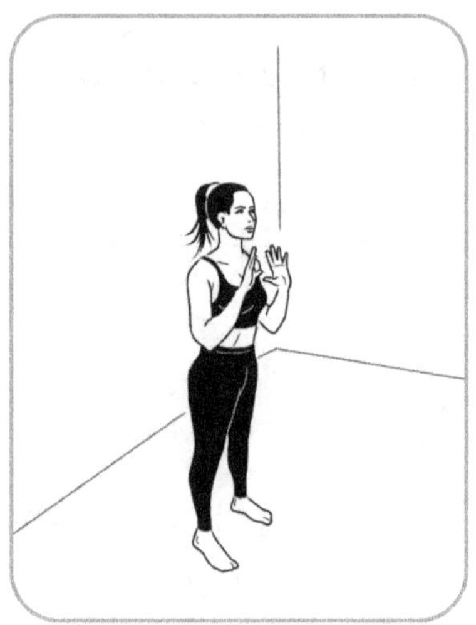

- Stand with your hands at chest level, keeping them as if you were holding a ball that you needed to throw. Take a deep inhale through the nose.

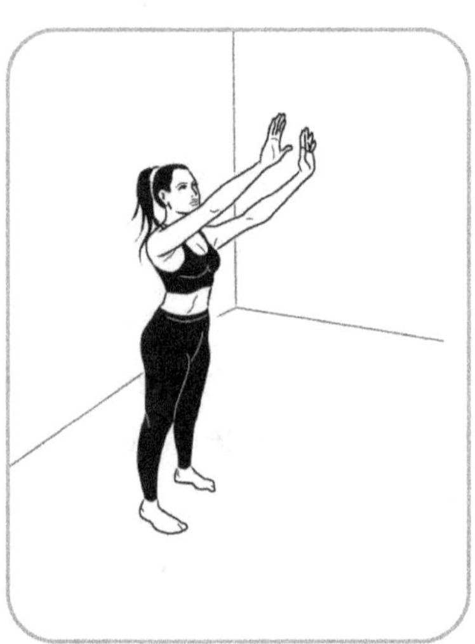

- Exhale fully through your nose and concentrate on expelling all of the negative energy within you. Push your arms forward and upward as if you were throwing the ball - imagine it as a "ball full of stress and bad experiences you have had recently".

- Return to the starting position and repeat the exercise for the specified number of repetitions.

Extra Tips:

This helps to 'push out' the trauma. Inhale while pulling your hands back, and exhale while pushing out. The pushing-out movement should be quick, while the return to the starting position should be slower.

STATIONARY SKIING

Great way to improve your full body awareness, strength, and cardio as well as releasing cortisol.

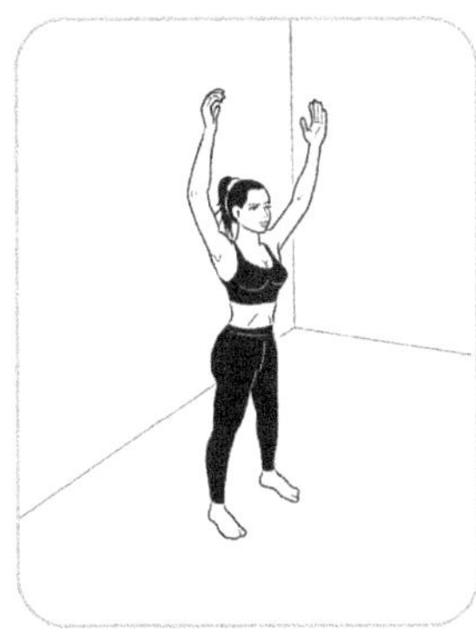

- Stand with your feet slightly wider than shoulder width apart and your arms extended above your head, as shown.

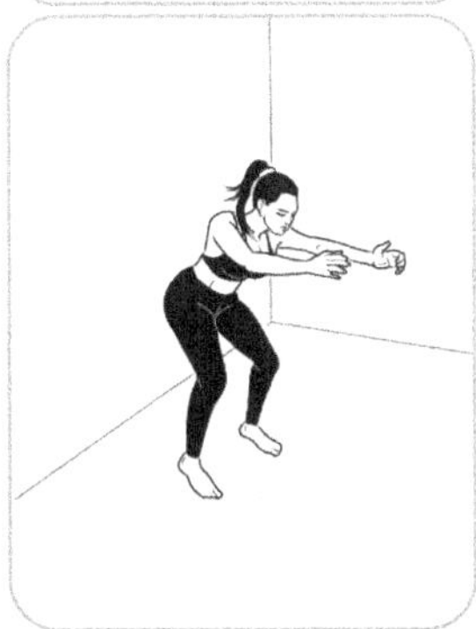

- Swing your hands down and bend your knees, bringing your buttocks back.

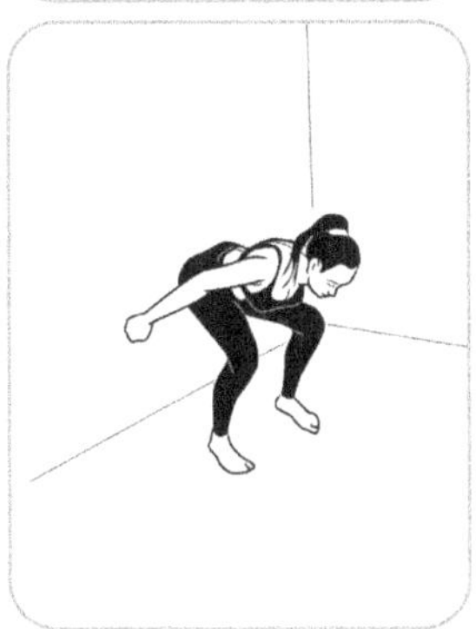

- Swing your hands backward and bend your knees close to 90 degrees, bringing your chest close to your thighs, as if you were skiing (Step 3).

- Return to the start position and repeat for the specified number of seconds.

Extra Tips:

The main focus here is to imagine you have all of the tension and anxiety in your hands. As you perform the movement, push it back and away from you. Exhale while performing the movement, then inhale when returning to the starting position.

The quicker you execute it, the more challenging it becomes. While three steps are demonstrated, the goal is to seamlessly perform them at such a rapid pace that the exercise defies easy categorization into distinct steps. In the 28-day plan, alternating between gentle and intense exercises is great for getting rid of toxins in your body, as well as releasing negative thoughts and emotional trauma.

PILLOW SLAM

Fantastic exercise to release negative energy quickly, and boost dopamine. It also helps dealing with passive aggressiveness.

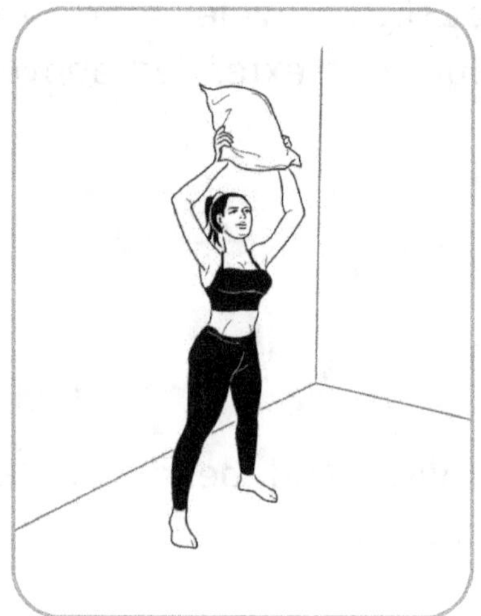

- Start by standing with your feet slightly wider than hip-width apart, and have a pillow over your head.

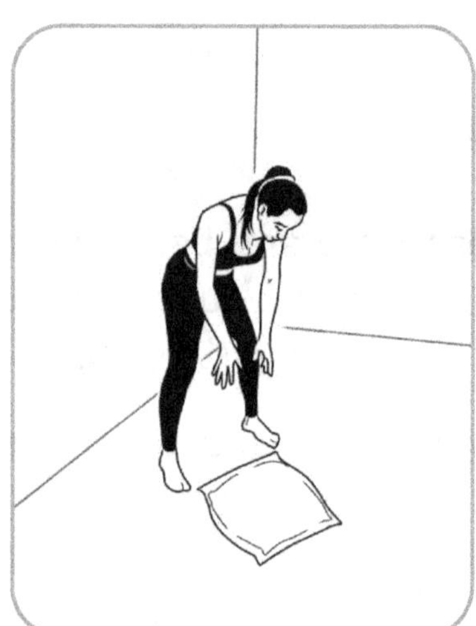

- From there, throw it on the floor, just in front of you.

- Then, pick it up again and repeat for the mentioned reps.

Extra Tips:

A great way to release stress. It is not necessary to slam the pillow down with maximal effort, but just enough to feel 'good' and release some stress. Doing it for a few reps will both tire you and make you feel emotionally better.

SIDE LUNGE AND EXTEND

Great exercise for upper body flexibility and strength. Breathing helps to release tension as you stretch over one side.

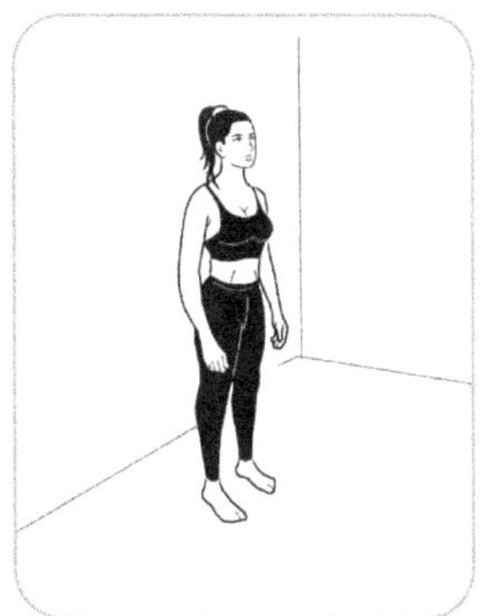

- Stand with your arms close to your body. Exhale gently before beginning to move.

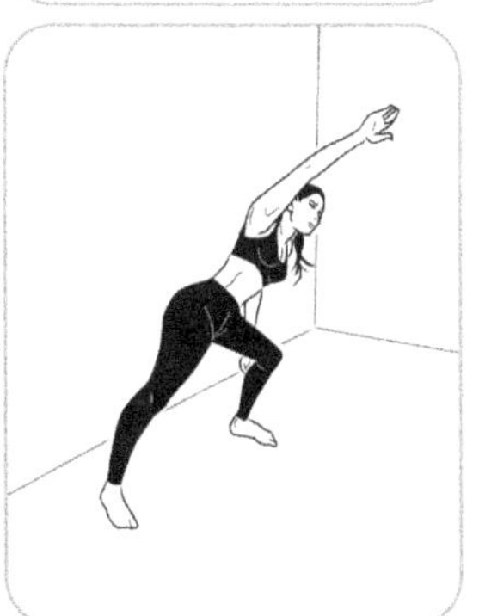

- Step your left foot to the left side, bending your left knee but keeping your right leg straight.

- Reach your right hand over your left side, as shown. Reach over with your right hand as high and wide as possible while leaning to the left. Hold the position for two seconds, exhaling completely.

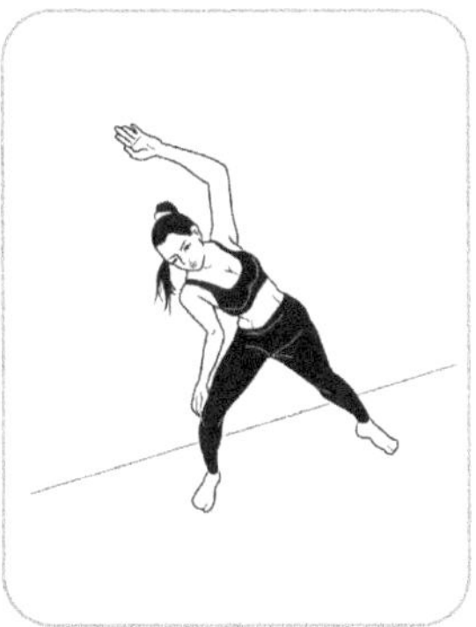

- Then, slowly return to the starting position, inhaling as you go, and repeat on the other side, performing the movement for the specified number of reps while alternating sides.

Extra Tips:

Control your breathing, take the exercise slowly, and concentrate on the muscles and your feelings. You might experience a burning sensation in your left quad and glute, as well as a stretch on the right side of your back. That's a common feeling while doing the exercise.

SEATED & CRAWLING EXERCISES
TRUNK REACH BACK

Great exercise to mobilize the upper back, shoulder, and lower back. Deep exhalation helps to relieve stress and tension.

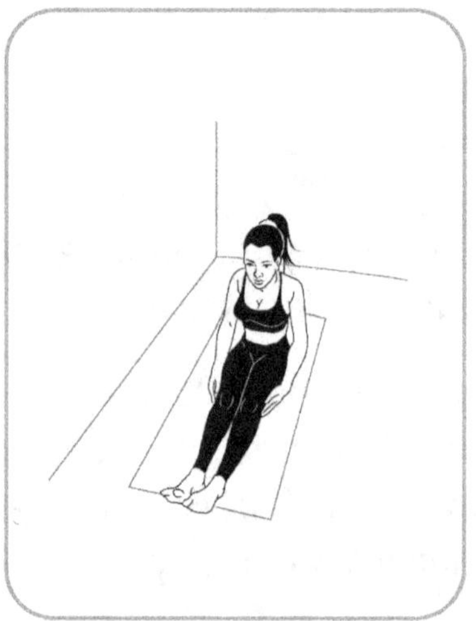

- Sit on the mat, legs straight in front of you.

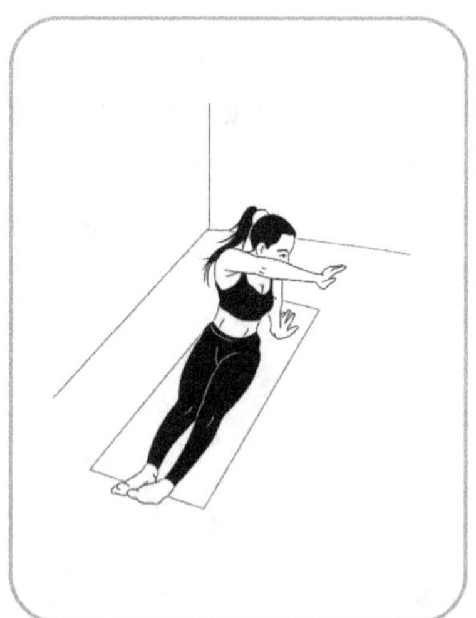

- Twist your back to the left, keeping your legs in the same position. Place your left hand on the floor and reach back with your right.

- Return to the starting position and repeat on the opposite side. Continue alternating the reps as specified in the 28-day plan.

Extra Tips:

I strongly recommend not doing the reps faster than they're supposed to be. Doing it slowly and controlled is more effective.

IN & OUT

Exercise to reduce anxiety and to increase presence. Reduces stress and improves neck, back, and knee health.

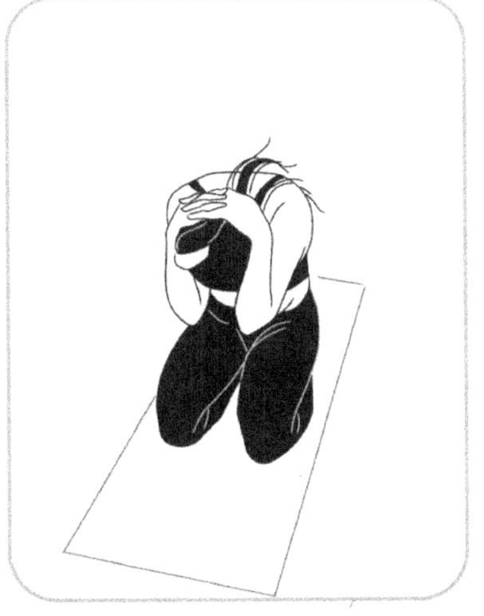

- Begin by sitting on your shins on the mat with a straight back. Place your hands behind your head, drop your chin to your collarbone, and keep your elbows closed as shown in the first image. Hold the position for two seconds.

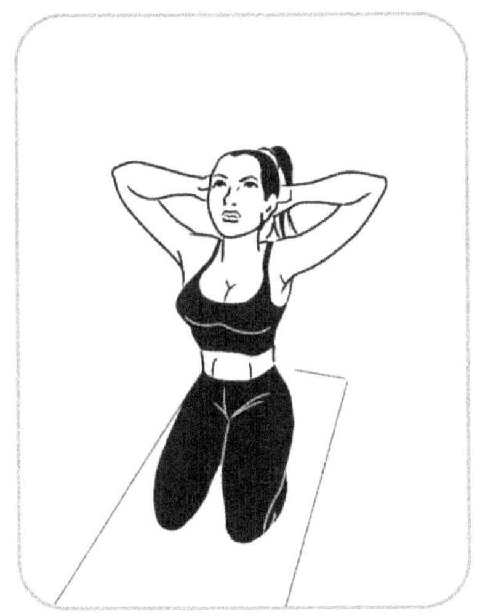

- Then, as you exhale, lift your head and extend your elbows and chest. Keep your hands against the back of your head. Hold this position for two seconds.

- Repeat the sequence for the specified number of times.

Extra Tips:

Make sure that as you perform the movement, you not only move your chin but also your spine, rounding it first (Step 1), and then extending it.

DOWNWARD CRAWLING

Excellent exercise for strengthening the lower body and core and improving coordination with your body.

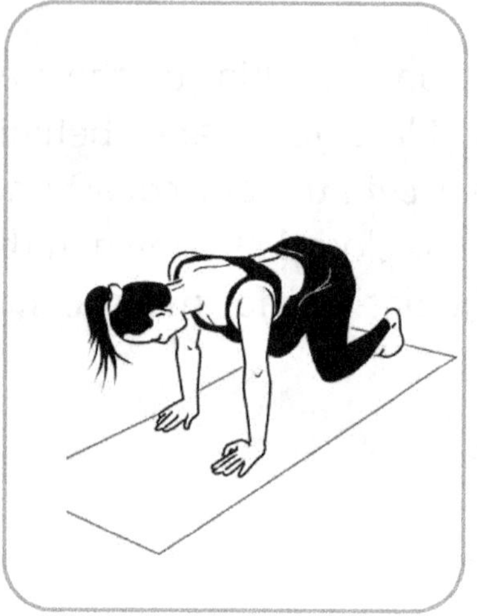

- Hands on the mat, arms straight, shoulders above your hands. Bend your knees to engage the quads, and elevate them so only your toes and hands are on the mat. Hold the position for 1 second and inhale through your nose.

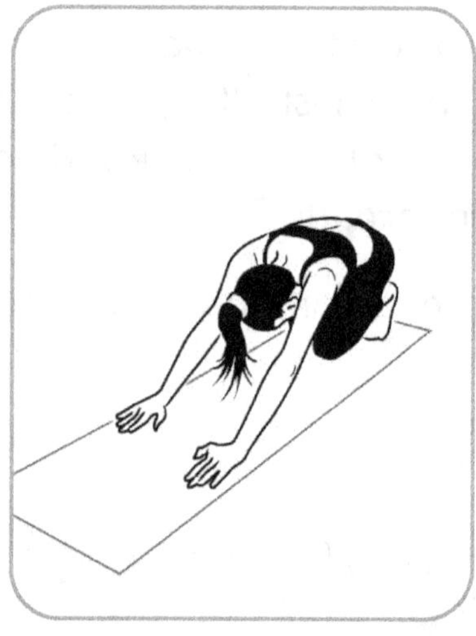

- Then, gently bring your hips closer to your heels to stretch your back while keeping your knees elevated and your arms straight, as shown in the second image. Exhale, and hold the position for one second.

- Finally, return to the starting position and repeat the movement for the number of times specified.

Extra Tips:

Perform the exercise slowly and with control over your body. It requires both strength and balance. Exhale deeply through your mouth to release any tension and make yourself feel present.

DOWNWARD DOG

Great exercise for flexibility and full-body harmony.

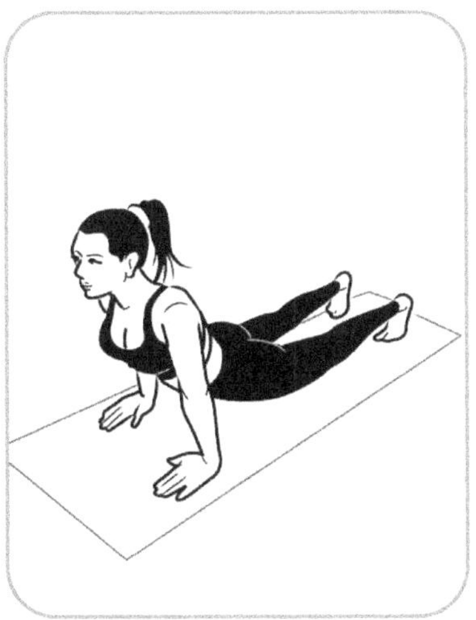

- Begin on the mat, with feet and hands on the ground. Maintain an elevated posture, with arms straight and chest up. This position requires both strength and flexibility. Inhale while in this position.

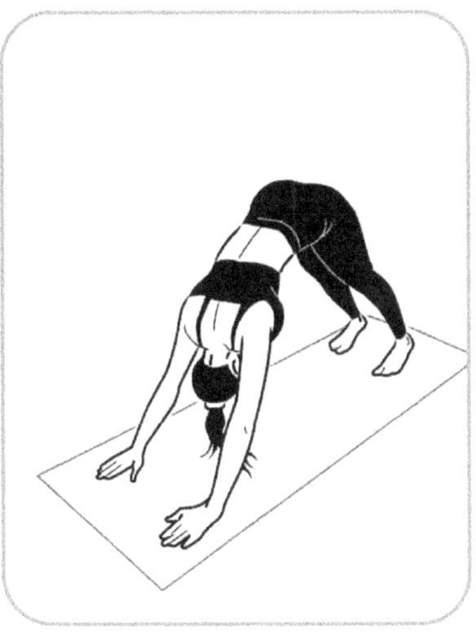

- Exhale as you lift your buttocks as far up as possible while keeping your feet and hands on the mat. Ensure that your legs and back are straight, as if you were attempting to form a triangle with the mat on the other side. Hold the position for one second.

- Return to the starting position and repeat for the specified number of times.

Extra Tips:

Concentrate on breathing and only stretch and relax the muscles that are required. Avoid tensing your body. This exercise is excellent for stretching your posterior chain, which is usually stiff due to a sedentary lifestyle.

If you feel too much stretch on the back of your leg as you lift your hips up in Step 2, you can slightly bend your knees. Over time, you'll be able to complete the exercise without bending them.

DYNAMIC PIGEON POSE

Effective exercise to enhance coordination, body control, and posture as well as releasing tension in the hips and back area.

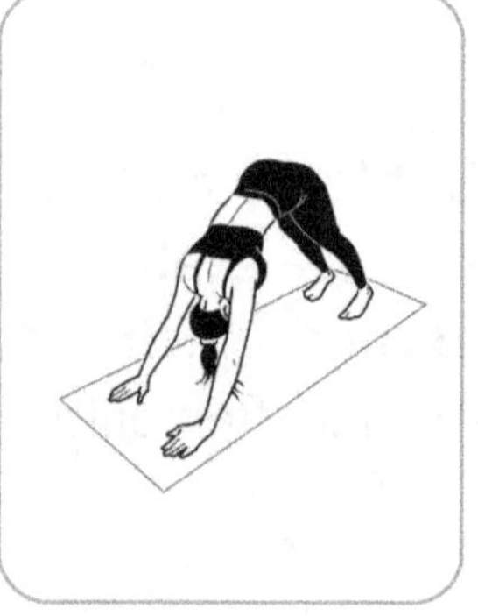

- Begin by placing your feet and hands on the mat and keeping your spine and legs straight. Lift your buttocks as much as possible. Keep your back straight. As you assume this position, you should feel a gentle stretch in your calves.

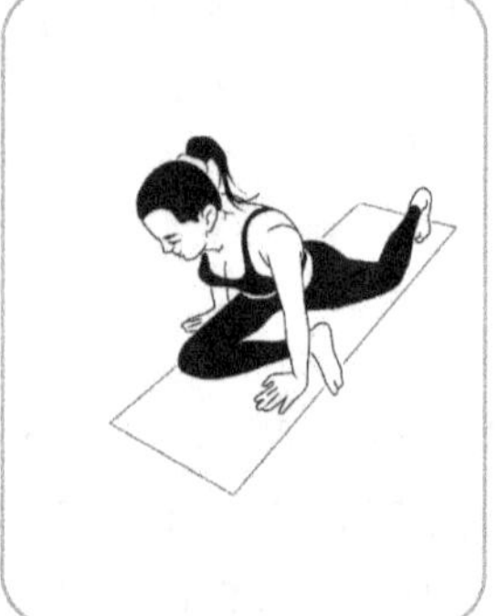

- Place the right knee on the floor and the right ankle between your left leg and left arm. Perform the movement slowly. You should feel a stretch in your right glute as you get into this position.

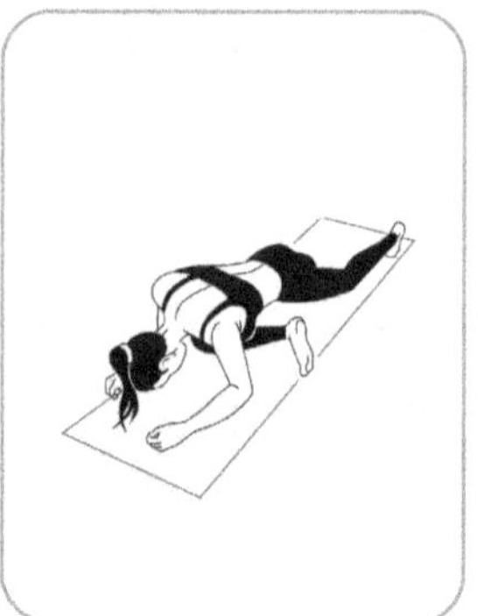

- Exhale fully and bring your chest close to the knee, using your arms for support if necessary, so that the lateral side of your thigh touches the mat. Hold the position for a full breath.

- Return to the starting position and repeat on the other side.

- Repeat it for the specified number of times, alternating sides.

Extra Tips:

If the Step 3 (last illustration) appears too difficult, simply try to bring your chest close to the floor. If you are unable to complete the task, that is fine. With practice, you'll improve your hip flexibility and make your movements more fluid by releasing unnecessary tension.

You should focus on each step and little movement of your body as you perform this exercise - there's no need to execute it fast.

90/90s

Effective exercise to release tension if you have stiff hips as well helping to get your cortisol levels regulated.

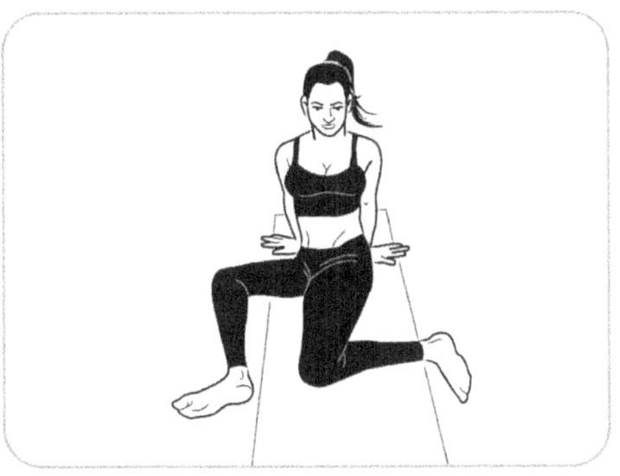

- Sit on the floor with your hands on the side of your waist on the floor (slightly behind if more comfortable), and your legs bent on one side with knees at 90°, as shown in the first image.

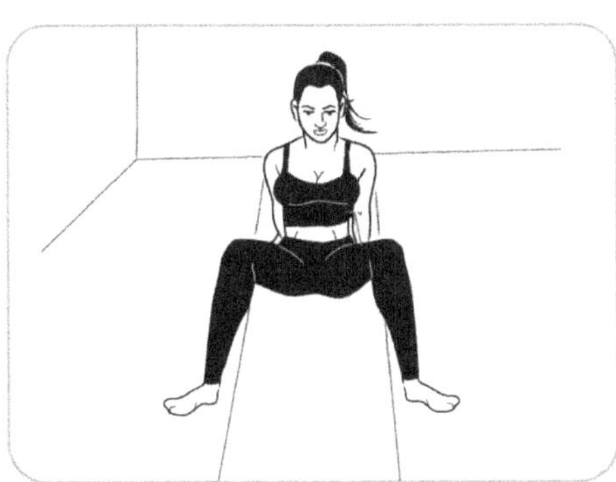

- Afterward, bring your legs back to the center position, paying attention to the movement of your hips, and maintain gentle and soft breathing through your nose.

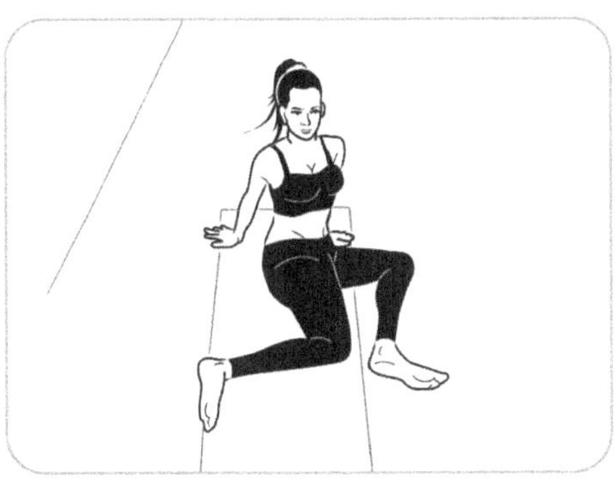

- Then, whilst keeping your trunk straight, move your hips to the other side.

- Perform it for the mentioned reps, alternating side to side.

Extra Tips:

It's common for people to tilt their trunk and round their spine when moving from side to side. Concentrate and make an effort to stay upright and centered with your trunk.

If you have any questions or doubts, feel free to contact me at zealyonsfitness@gmail.com, and I'll be happy to assist you the best I can about somatic exercises and workouts!

ANTI-STRESS PLANK

Great for both strength and mobility in your hips and core area.

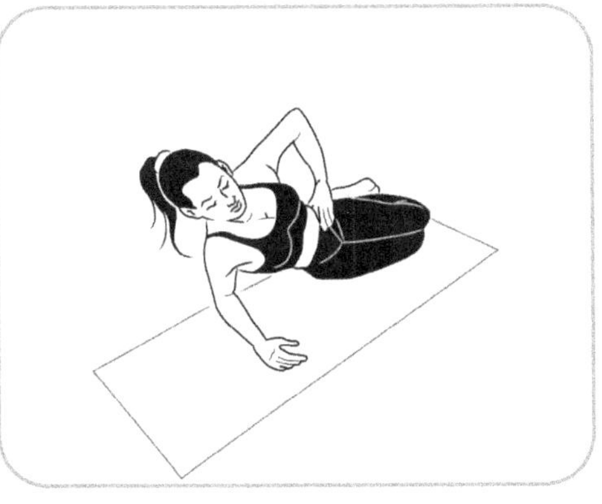

- Lay down on one side with your right forearm and the outside of the right knee on the floor.

- Then, slightly move your hips down, as shown.

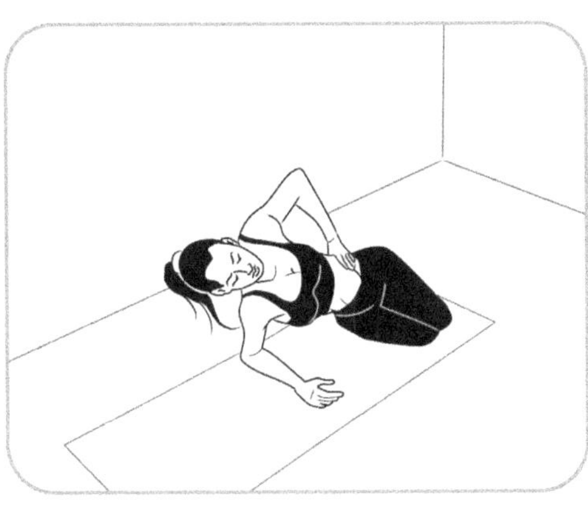

- From there, raise the hips slightly; although the range of motion may not be extensive, you will notice the impact as you execute the movement.

- Repeat the position for the mentioned seconds. Lastly, repeat the movement on the other side.

Extra Tips:

If it feels too easy, overtime you will be able to do it with your feet touching the floor instead of your knees. That would be very advanced and work many muscles of your body.

SEATED SIDE REACH

Good activation of the psoas as well as releasing stiffness on your back often caused by unnecessary stress.

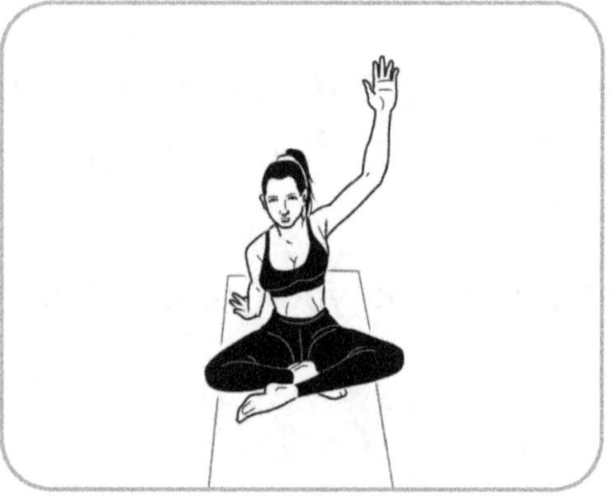

- Start by sitting on the floor crossing your legs. Place your right hand on the floor behind you (and slightly to the side) for assistance and balance, whilst having your left arm lifted in the air.

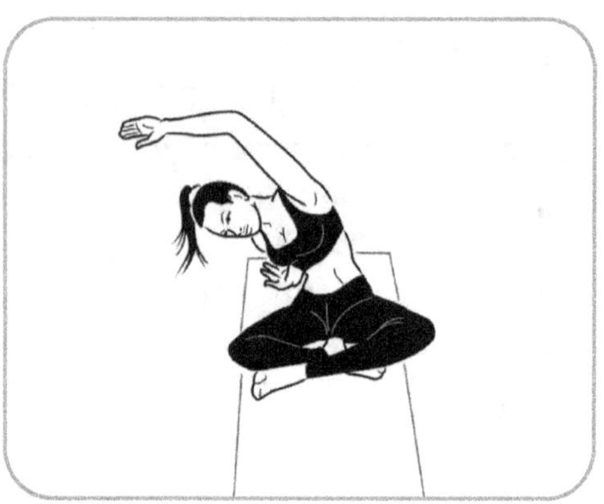

- From this position, move the left arm to the right side to stretch the left side of the back. Hold it for 2 seconds.

- Then, come back to the starting position, and repeat to the opposite side.

- Perform the movement for the mentioned reps, alternating the sides.

Extra Tips:

Make sure to exhale deeply from your mouth as you stretch on the side. Doing this for a few reps on each side will make you feel fantastic and lighter. As you come back into the starting position, inhale gently through your nose.

TOP POINT & FLEX PULSES

Great for connecting with your body, shaking your emotional state and improving mobility with simple exercise.

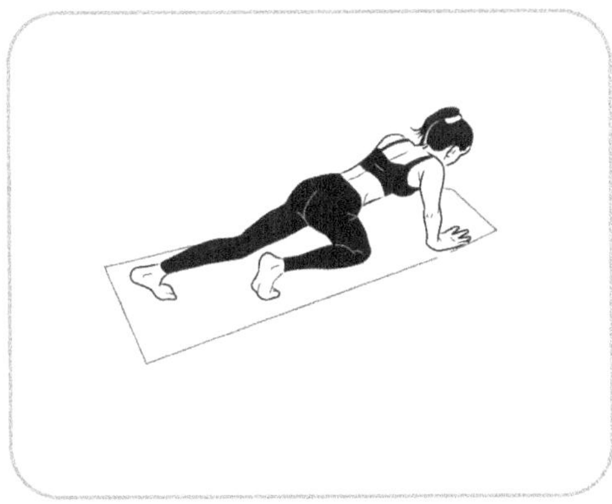

- Start in a half plank position with your arms straight with hands on the floor, and your right knee on the floor - see the illustrations for further assistance.

- From there, bring your hips slightly back, as shown.

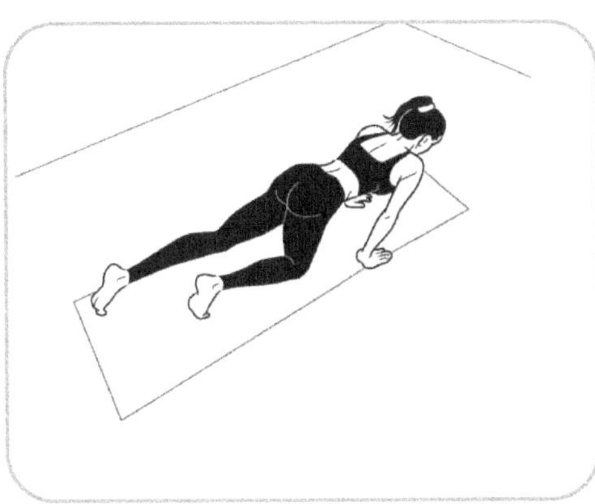

- Then, quickly by pulsing with your toes, move forward, almost extending your left leg straight.

- Keep repeating this sequence for the mentioned seconds. Then, repeat it on the other side.

Extra Tips:

Make sure not to hold your breath and keep inhaling and exhaling as you perform this movement.

28-DAY PLAN
HOW TO READ THE 28 DAY PLAN

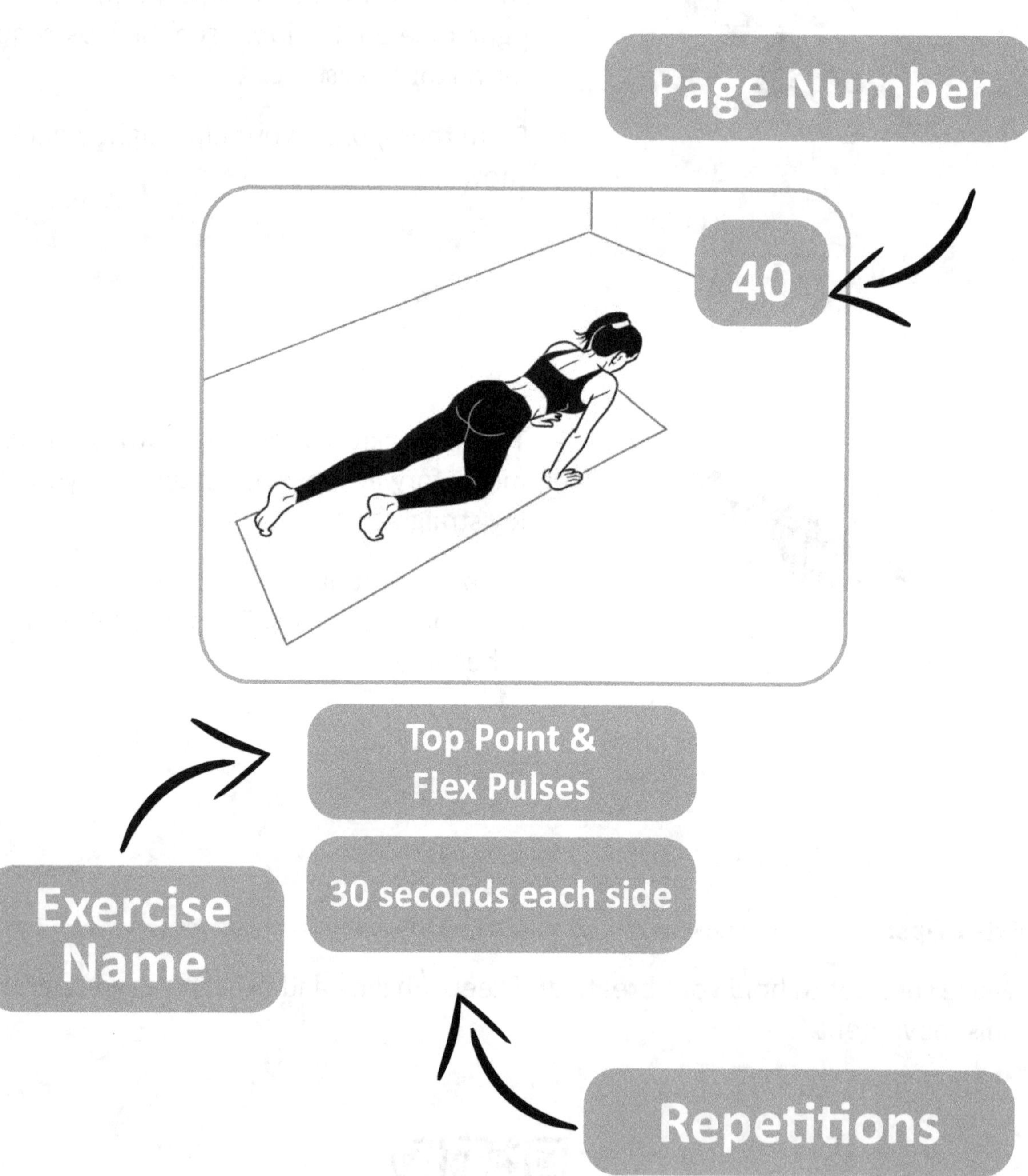

Day 1 - Repeat it twice.

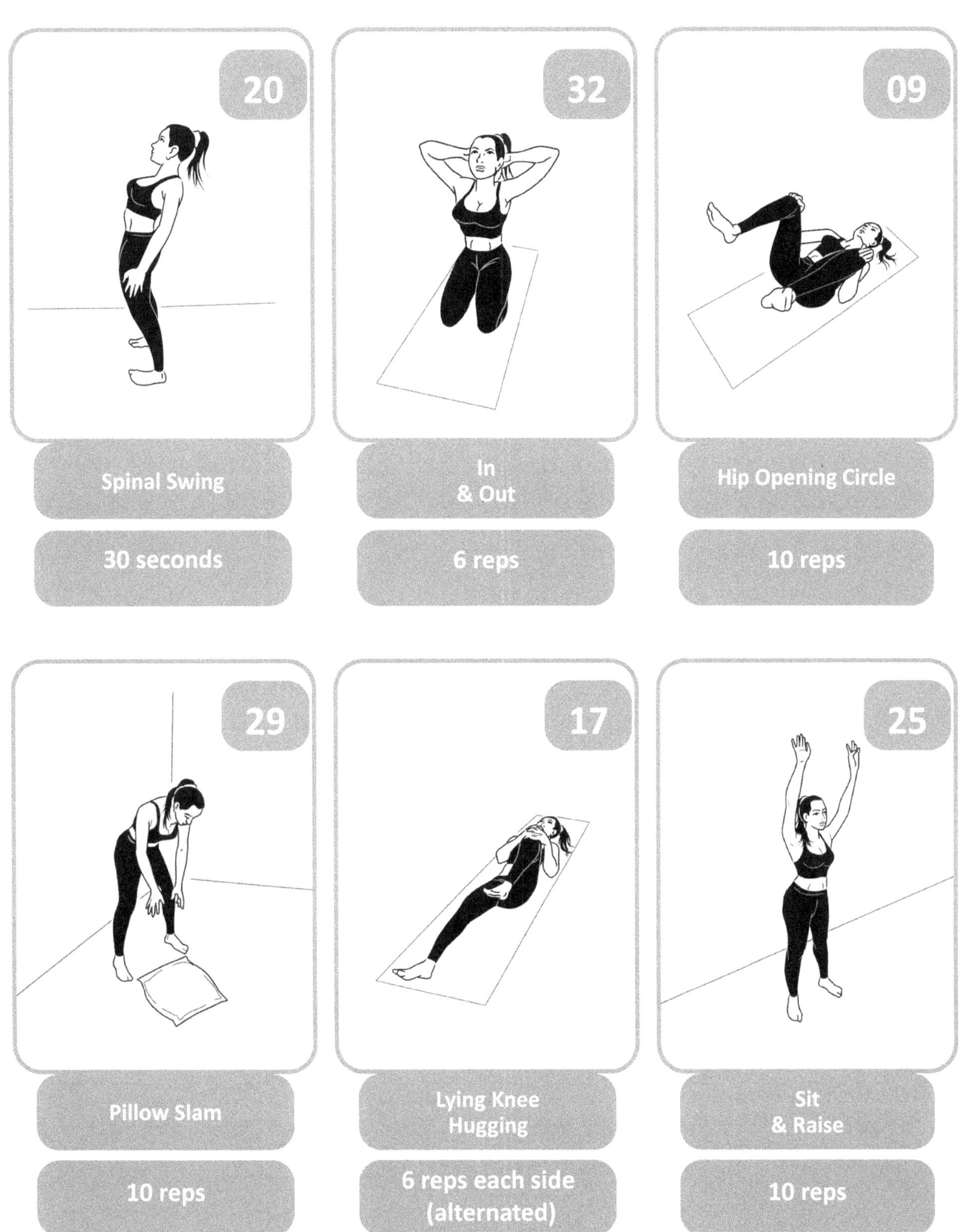

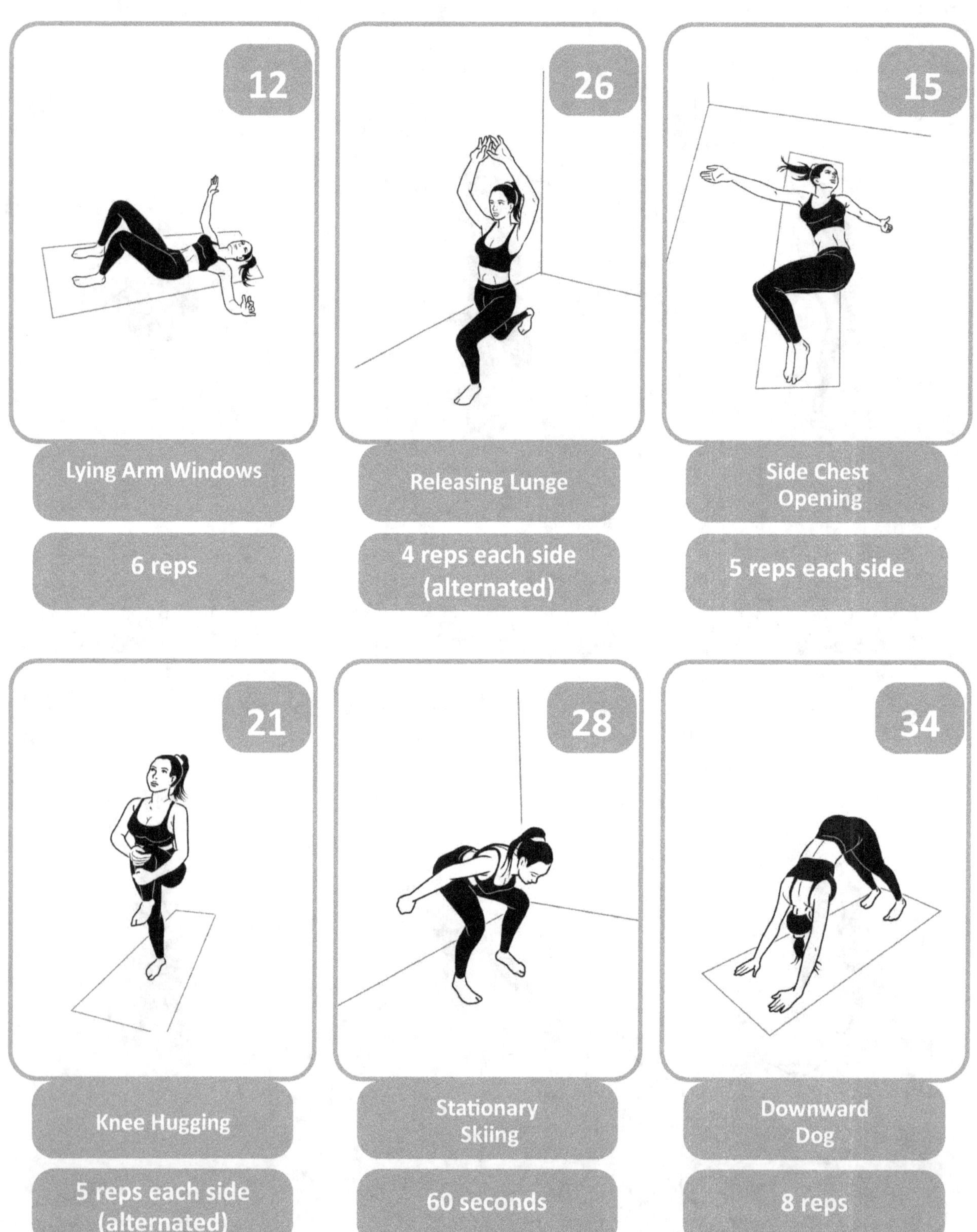

12	26	15
Lying Arm Windows	Releasing Lunge	Side Chest Opening
6 reps	4 reps each side (alternated)	5 reps each side
21	28	34
Knee Hugging	Stationary Skiing	Downward Dog
5 reps each side (alternated)	60 seconds	8 reps

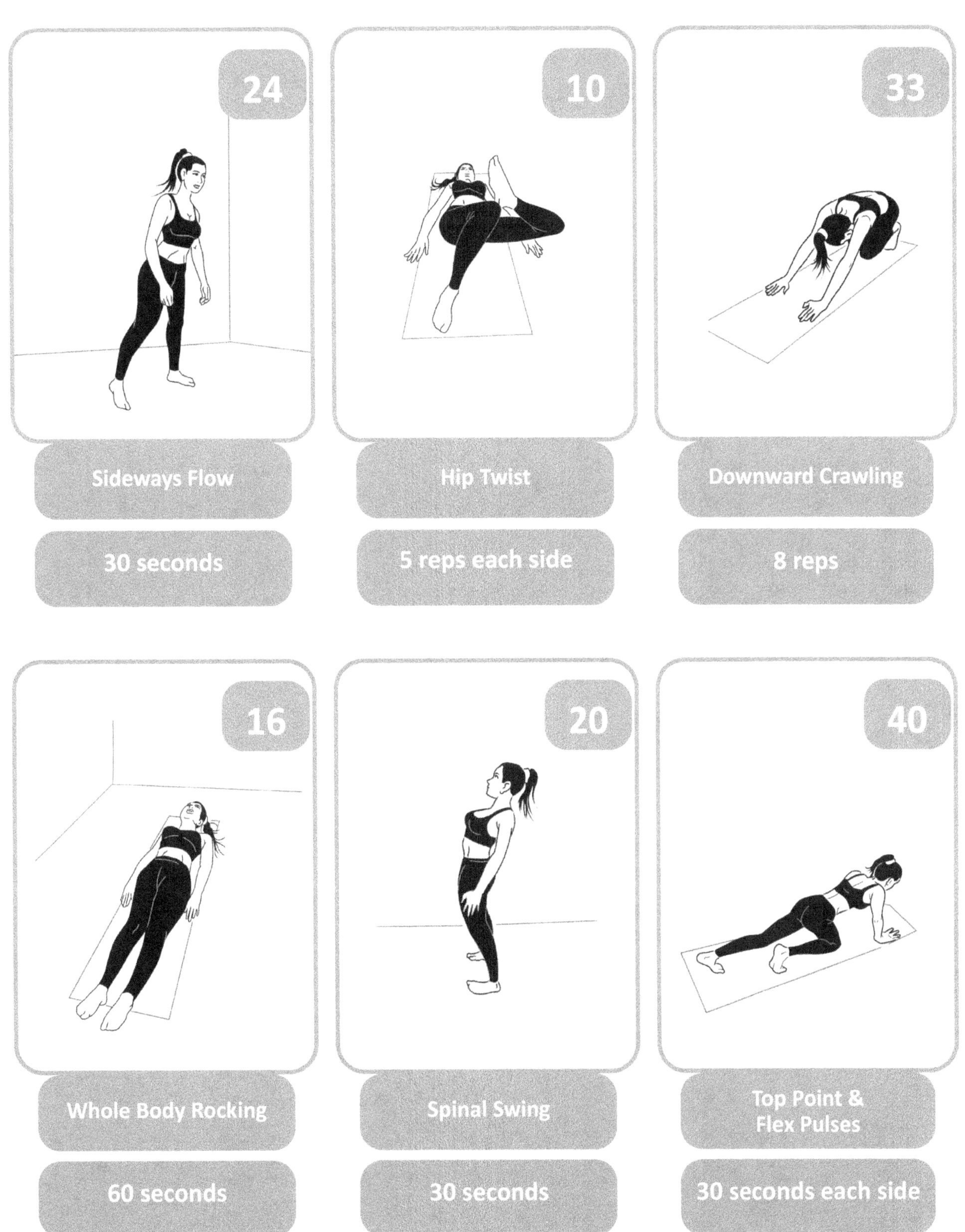
24
Sideways Flow
30 seconds

10
Hip Twist
5 reps each side

33
Downward Crawling
8 reps

16
Whole Body Rocking
60 seconds

20
Spinal Swing
30 seconds

40
Top Point &
Flex Pulses
30 seconds each side

Day 4 - Repeat it twice

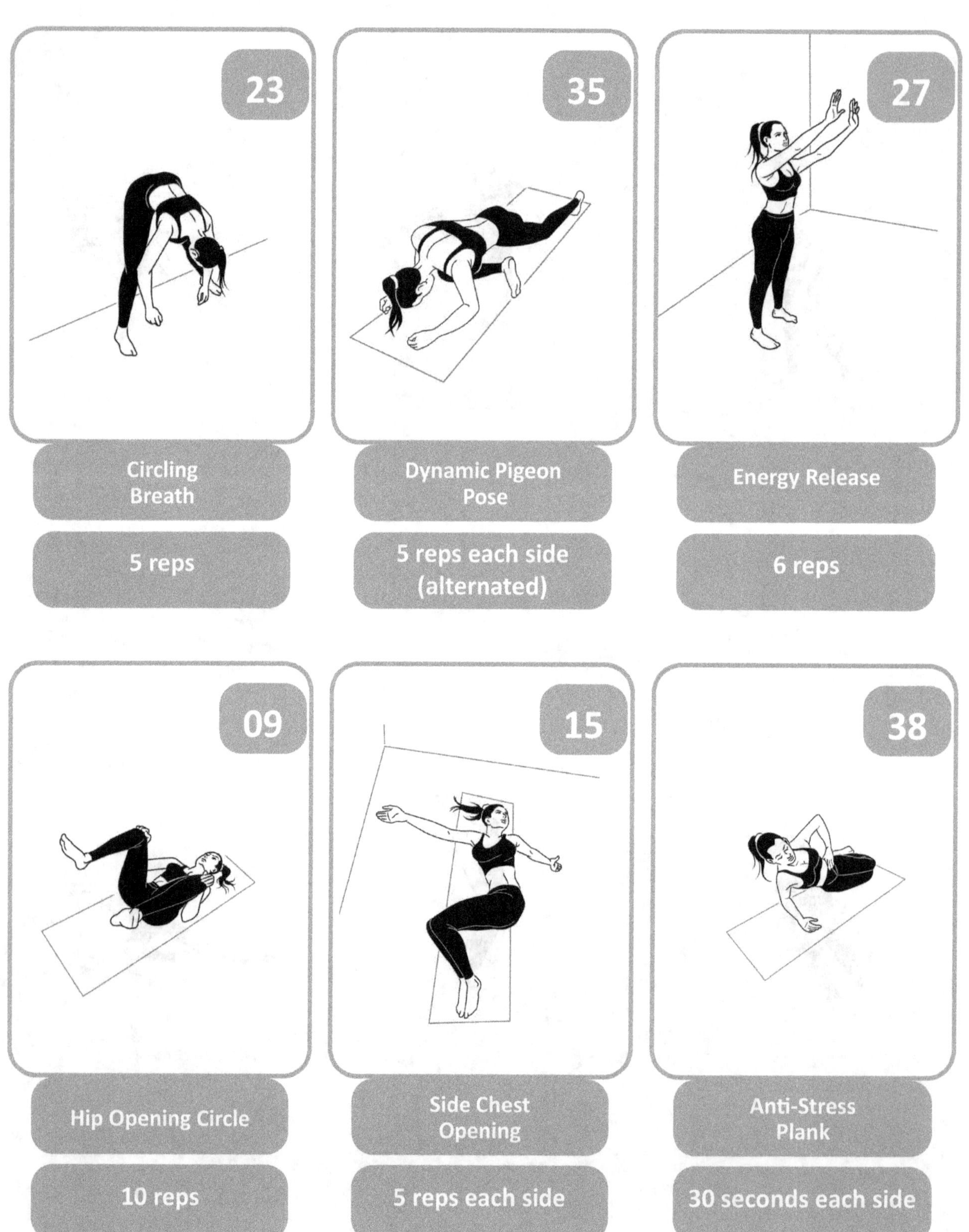

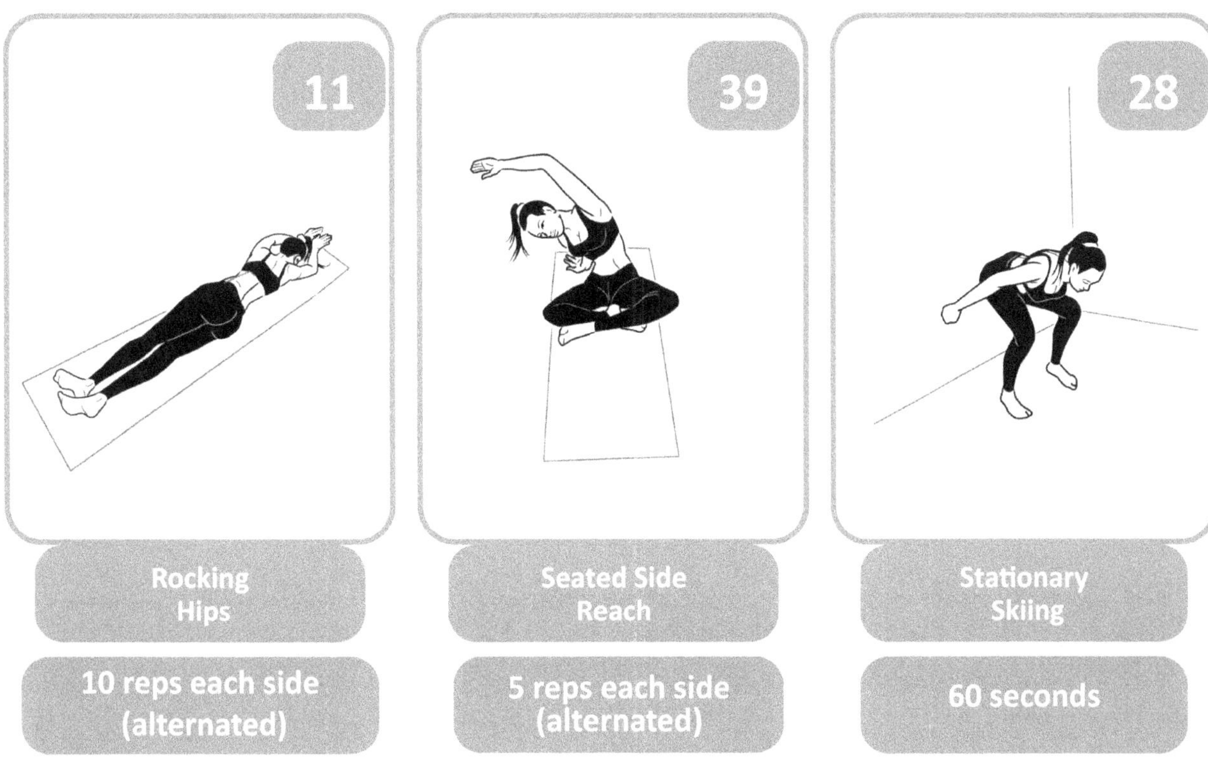

11
Rocking
Hips
10 reps each side
(alternated)
39
Seated Side
Reach
5 reps each side
(alternated)
28
Stationary
Skiing
60 seconds

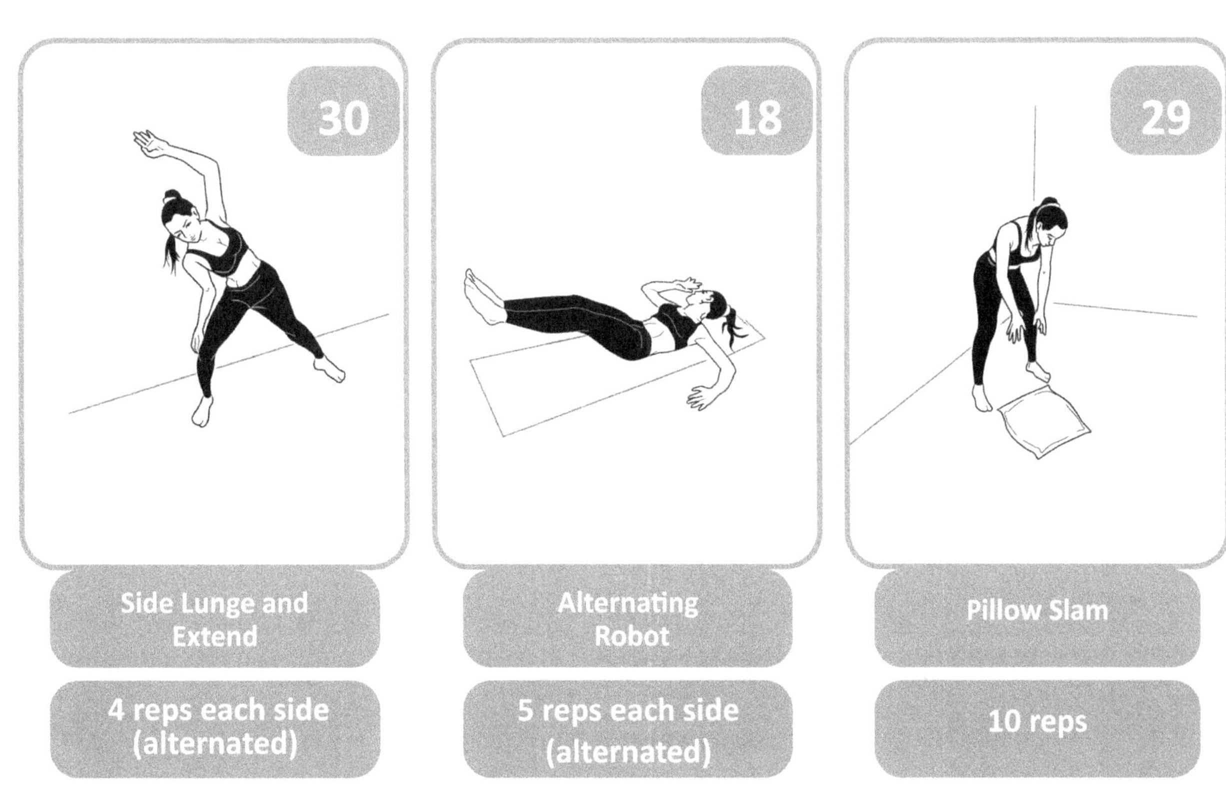

30
Side Lunge and
Extend
4 reps each side
(alternated)
18
Alternating
Robot
5 reps each side
(alternated)
29
Pillow Slam
10 reps

Day 6 - Repeat it twice.

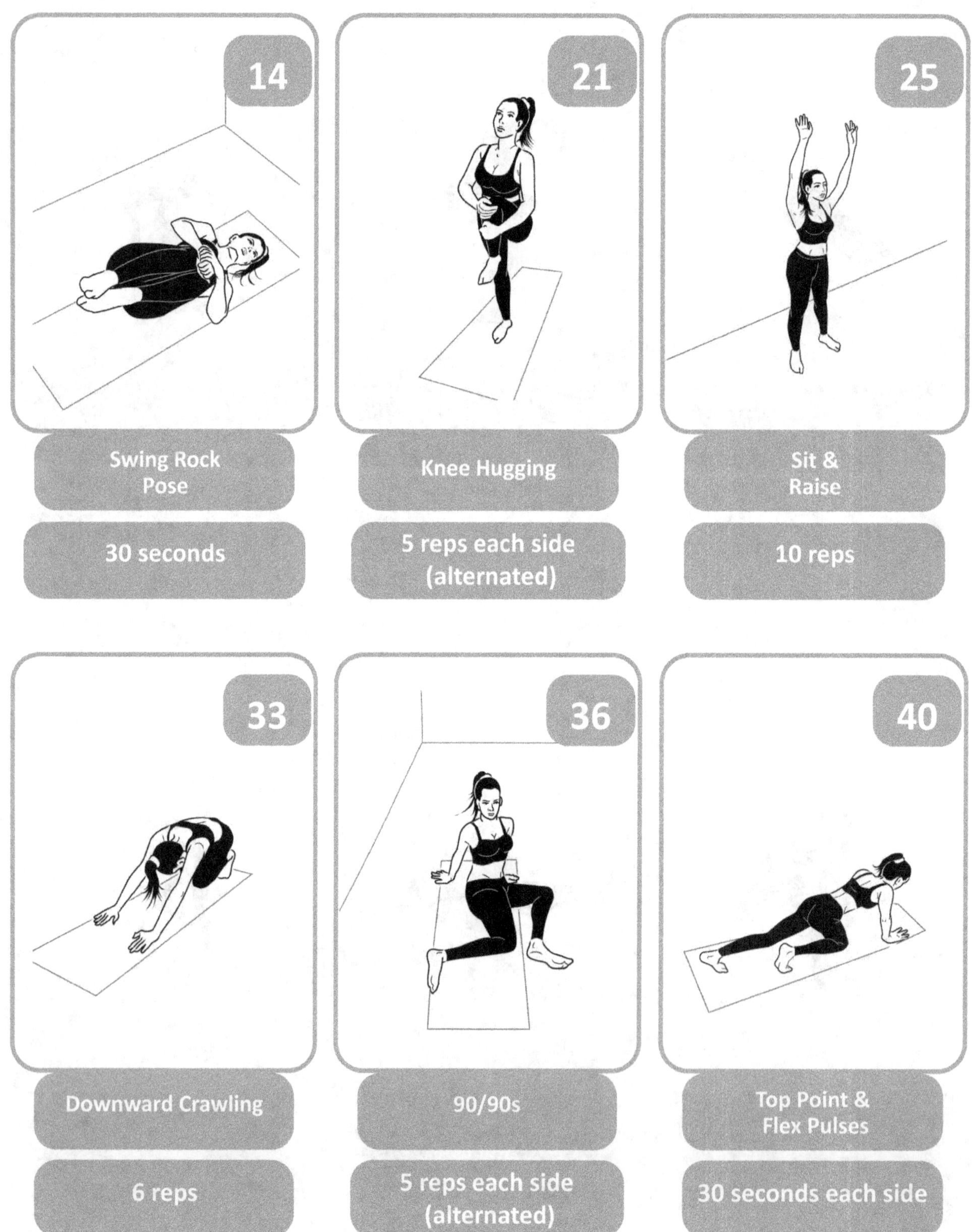

Day 7 - Repeat it twice.

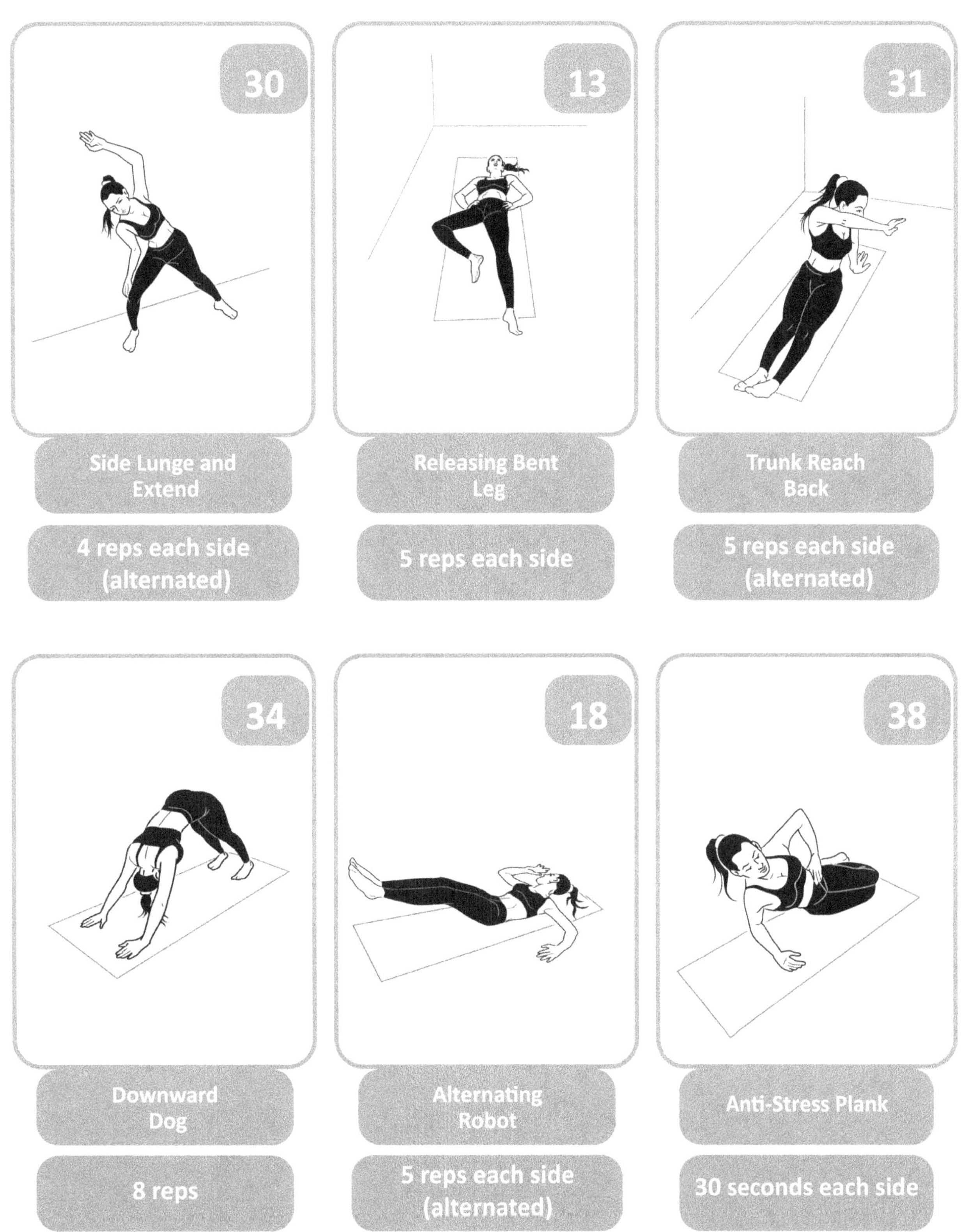

Day 8 - Repeat it twice.

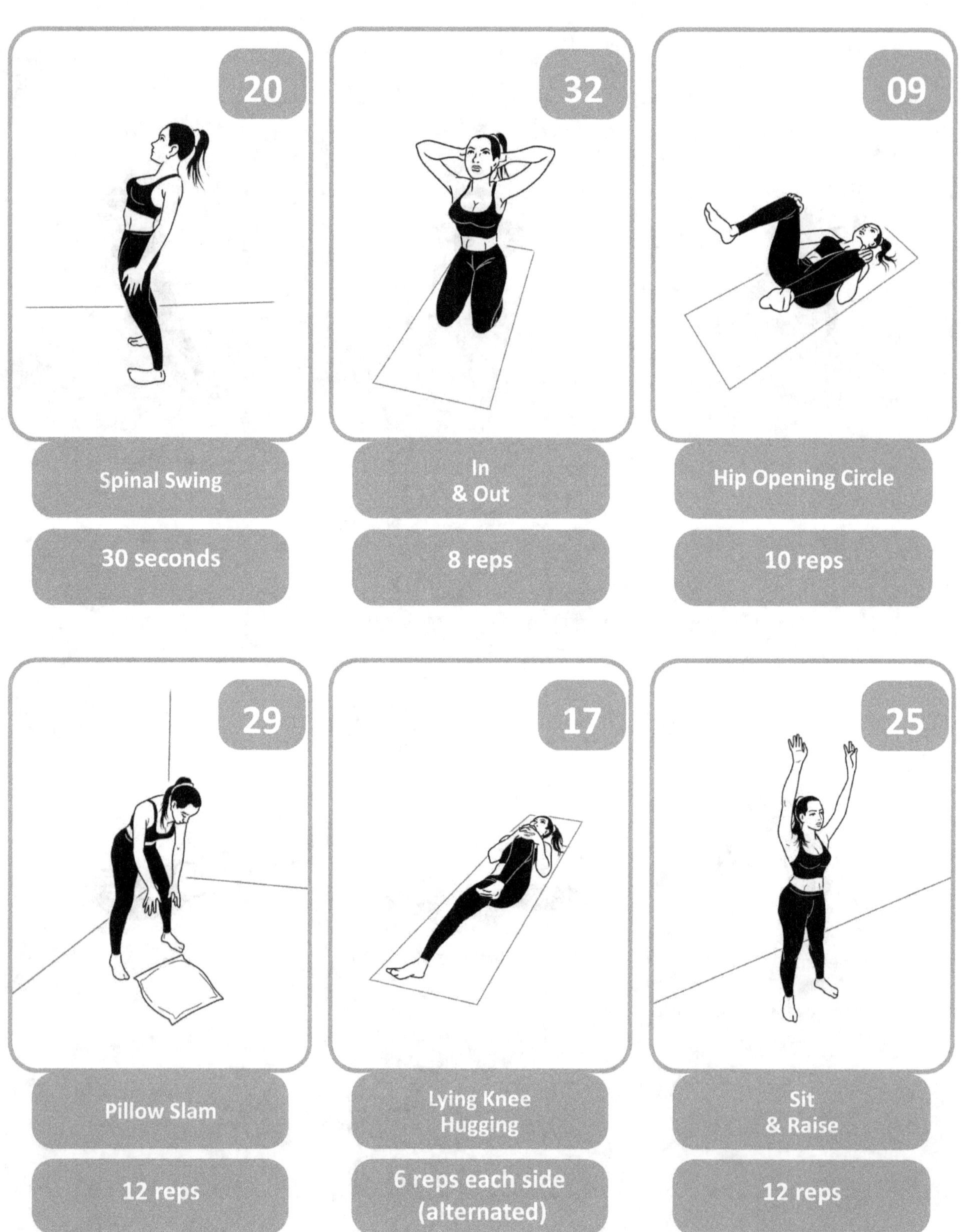

Day 9 - Repeat it three times.

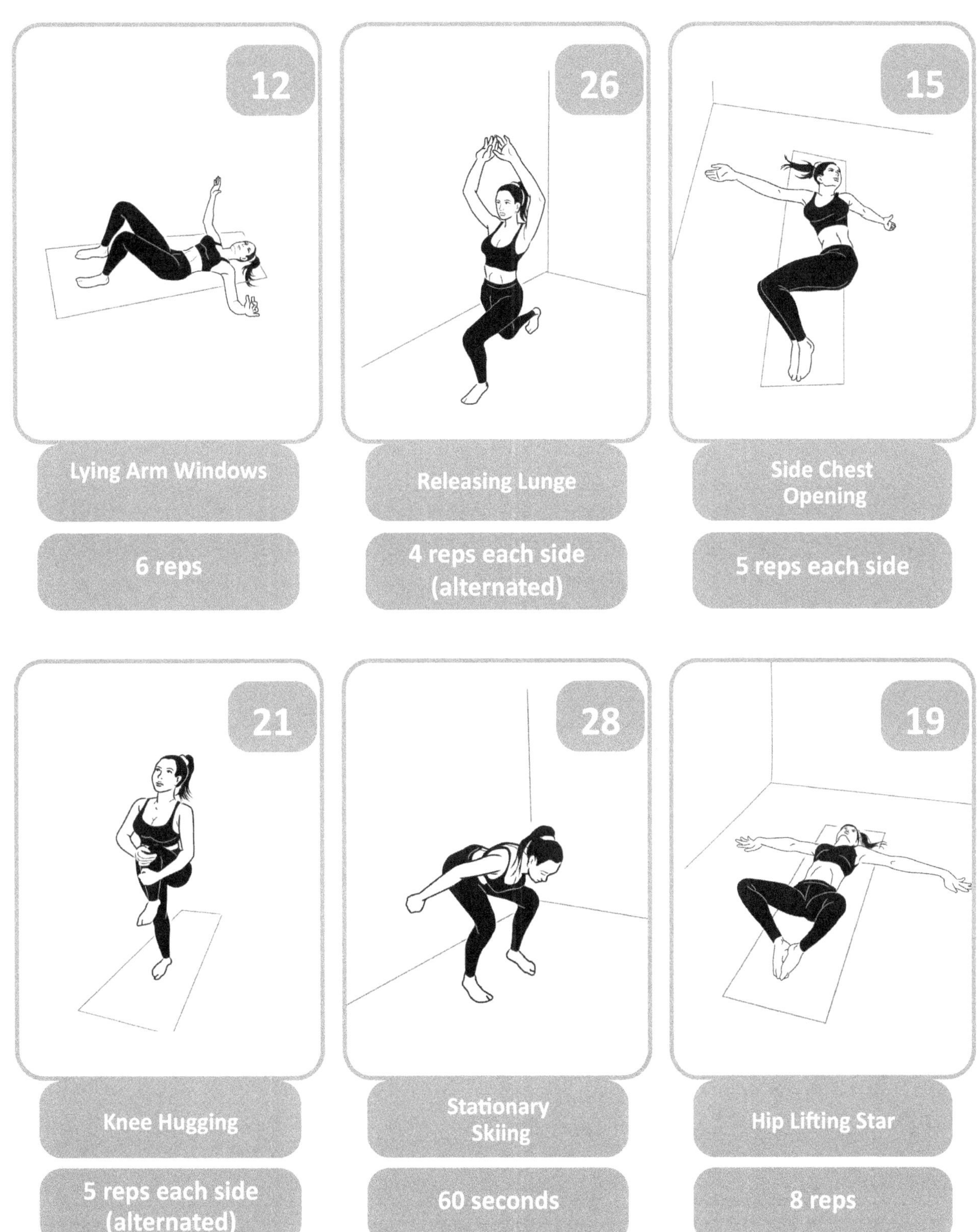

12	26	15
Lying Arm Windows	Releasing Lunge	Side Chest Opening
6 reps	4 reps each side (alternated)	5 reps each side

21	28	19
Knee Hugging	Stationary Skiing	Hip Lifting Star
5 reps each side (alternated)	60 seconds	8 reps

Day 10 - Repeat it twice.

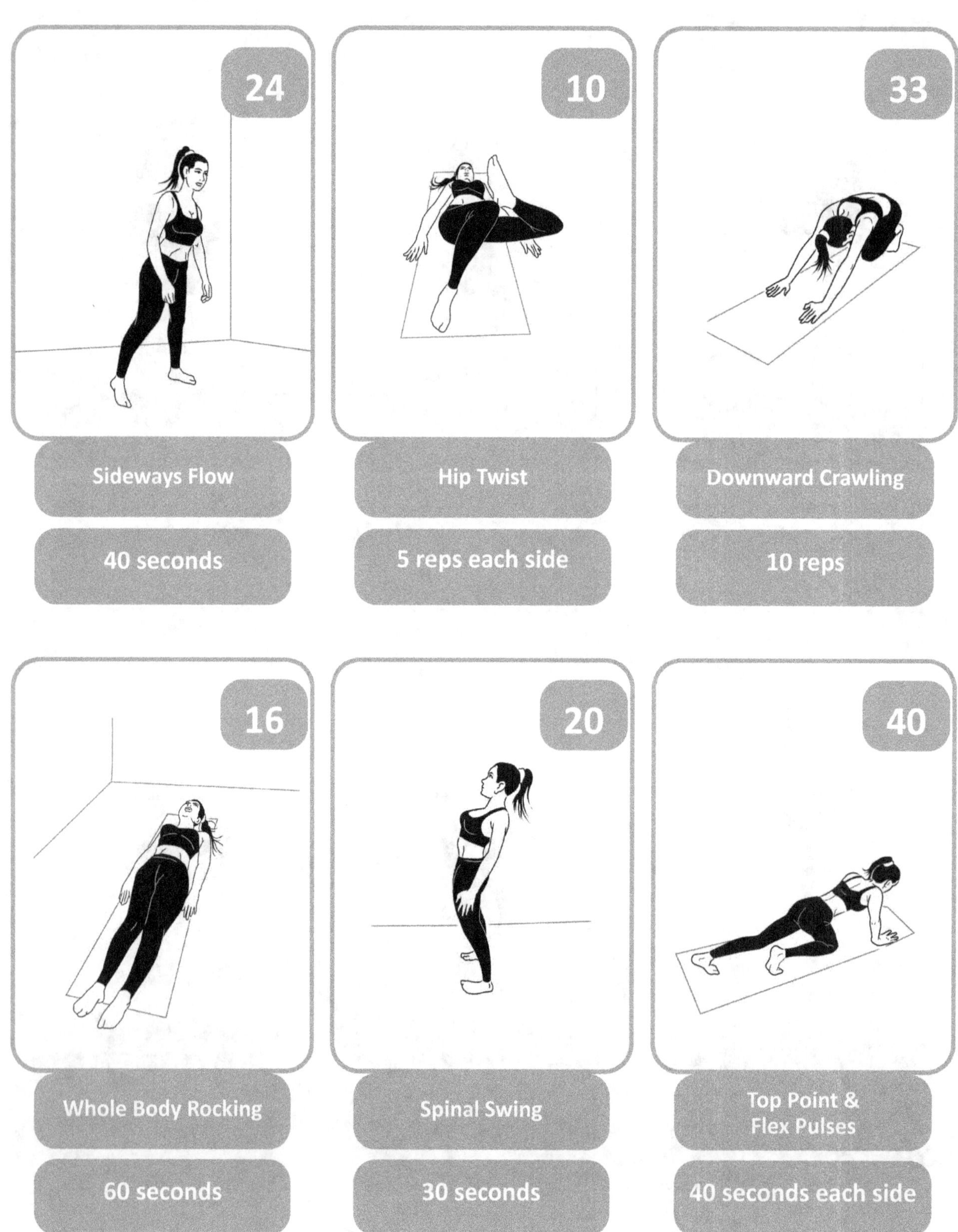

Day 11 - Repeat it three times

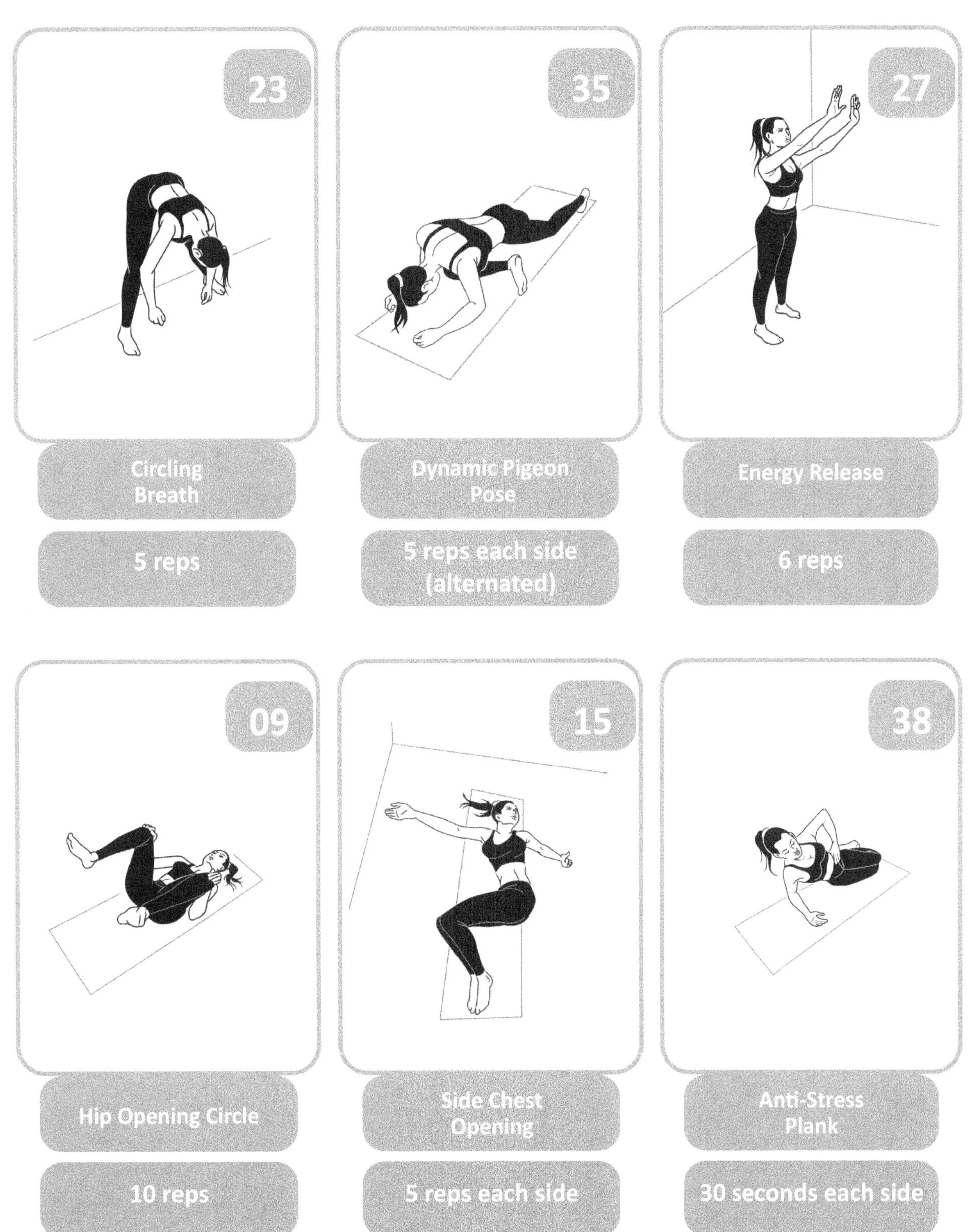

Day 12 - Repeat it twice.

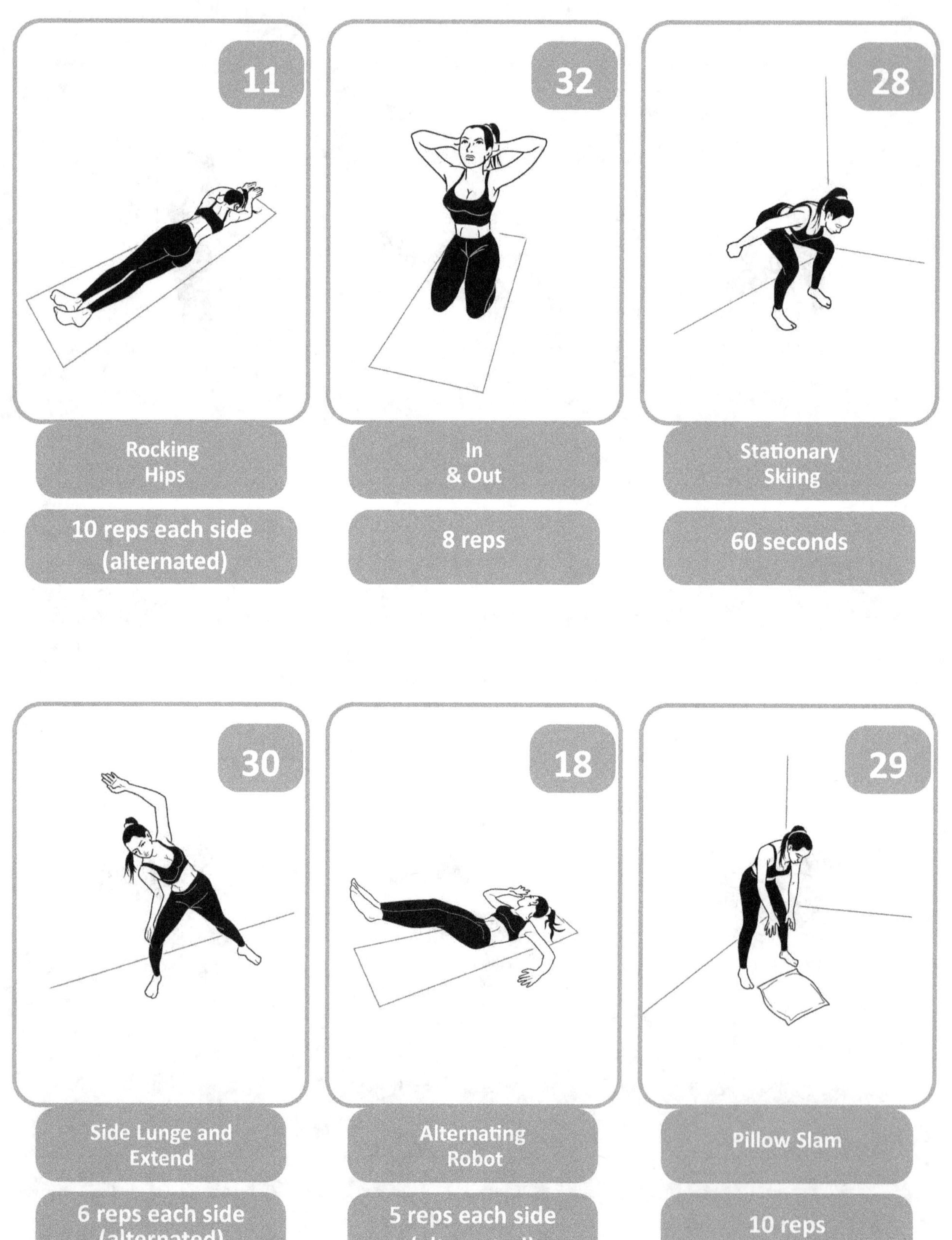

Day 13 - Repeat it three times.

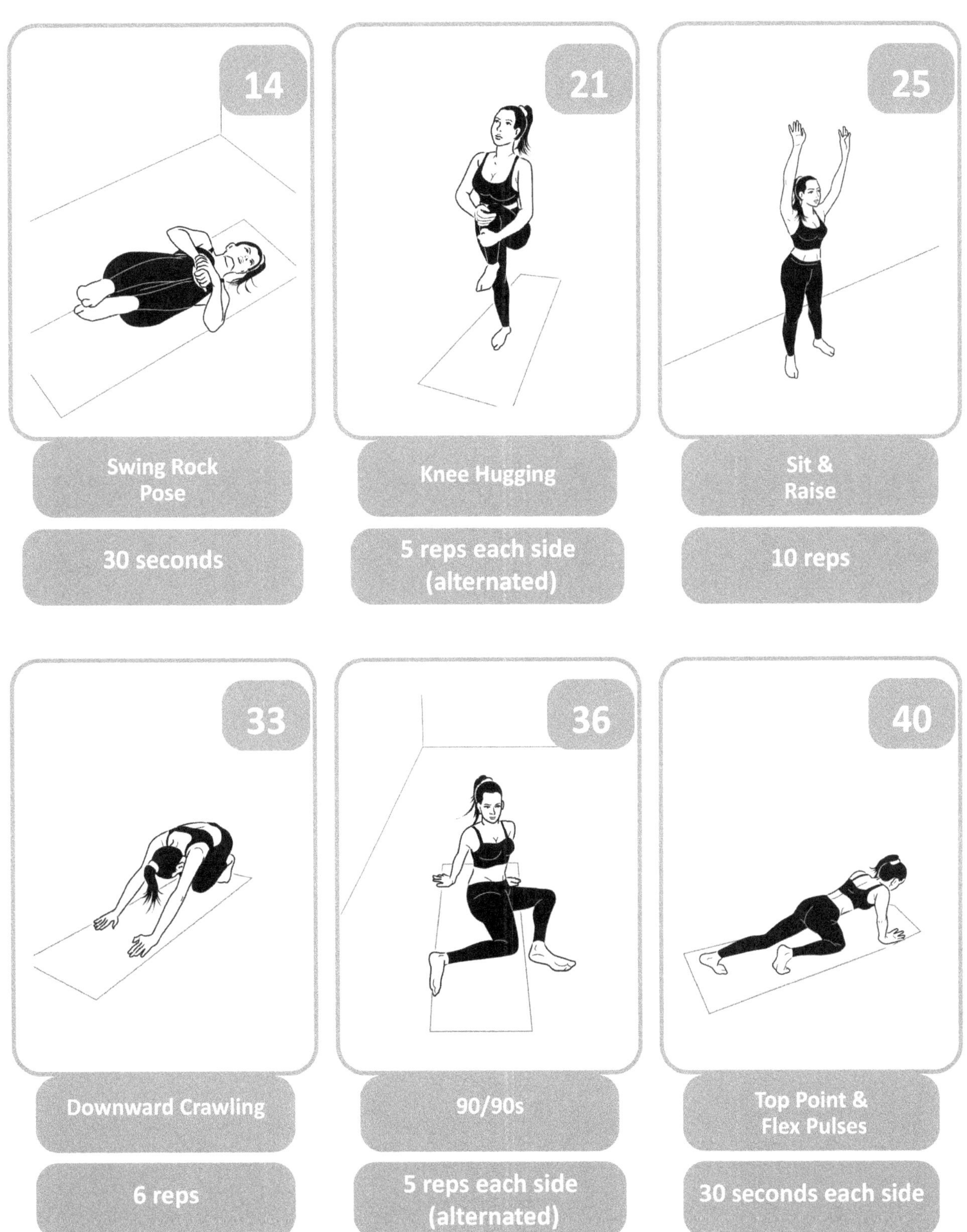

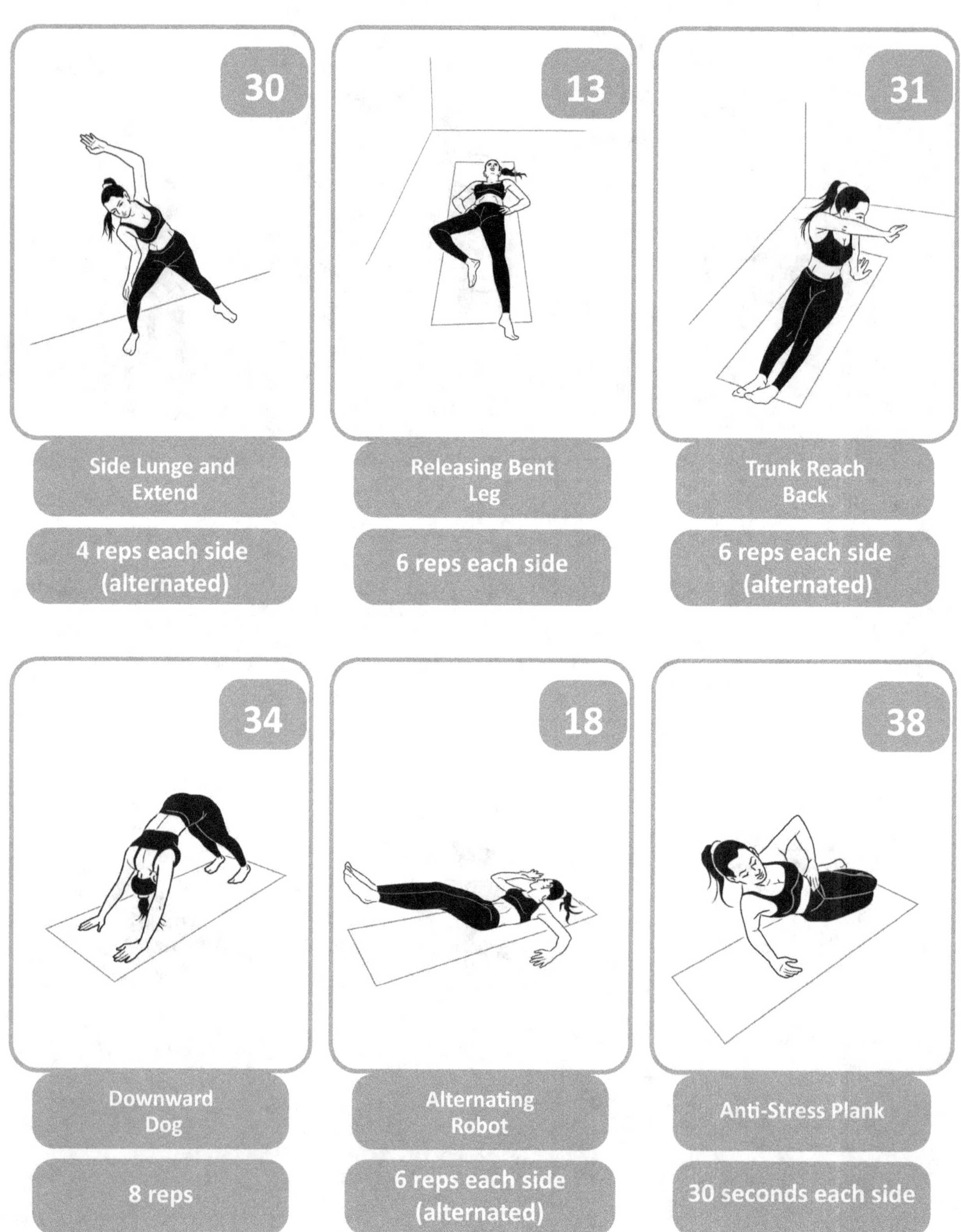

30
Side Lunge and Extend
4 reps each side (alternated)

13
Releasing Bent Leg
6 reps each side

31
Trunk Reach Back
6 reps each side (alternated)

34
Downward Dog
8 reps

18
Alternating Robot
6 reps each side (alternated)

38
Anti-Stress Plank
30 seconds each side

Day 15 - Repeat it three times.

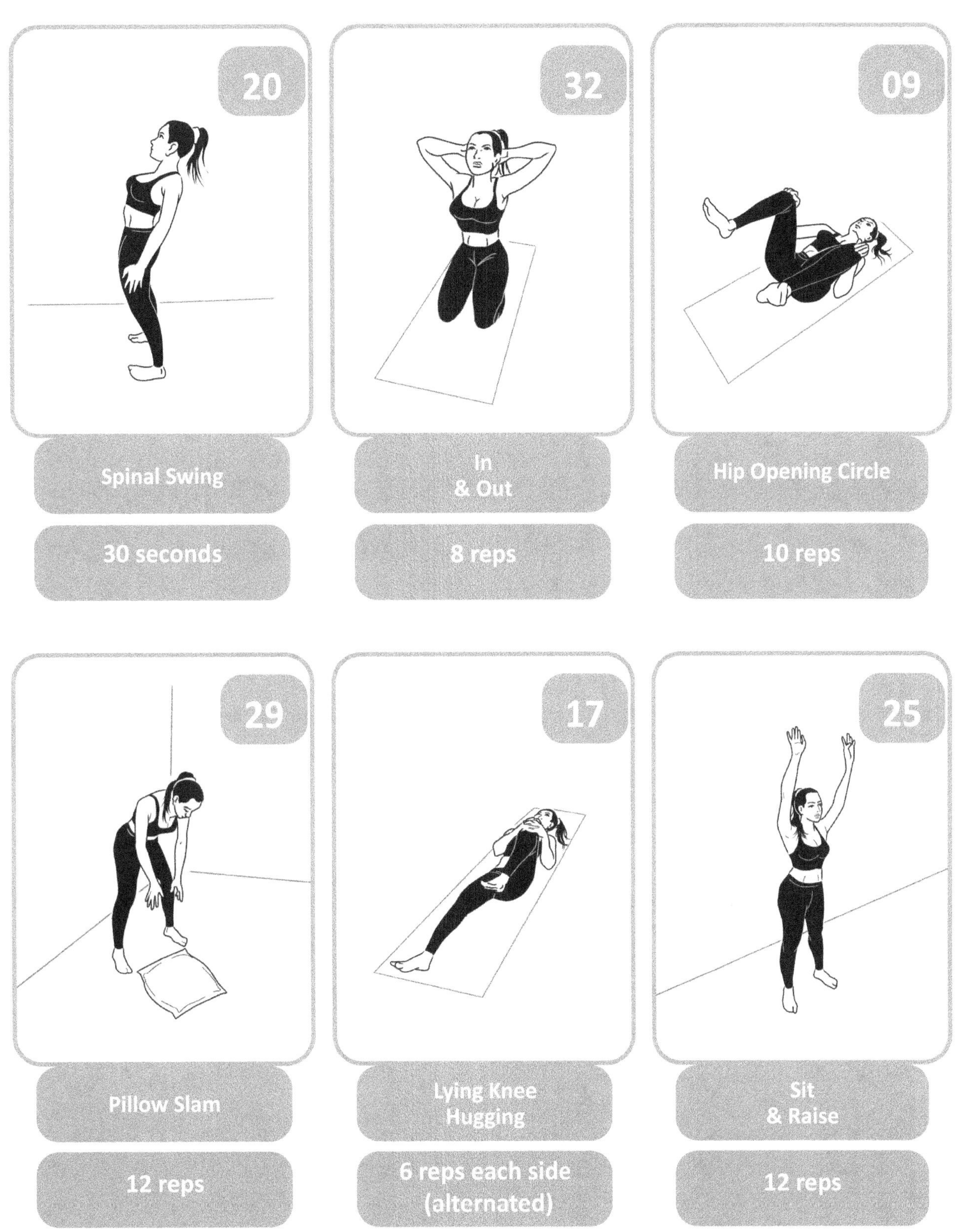

Day 16 - Repeat it three times.

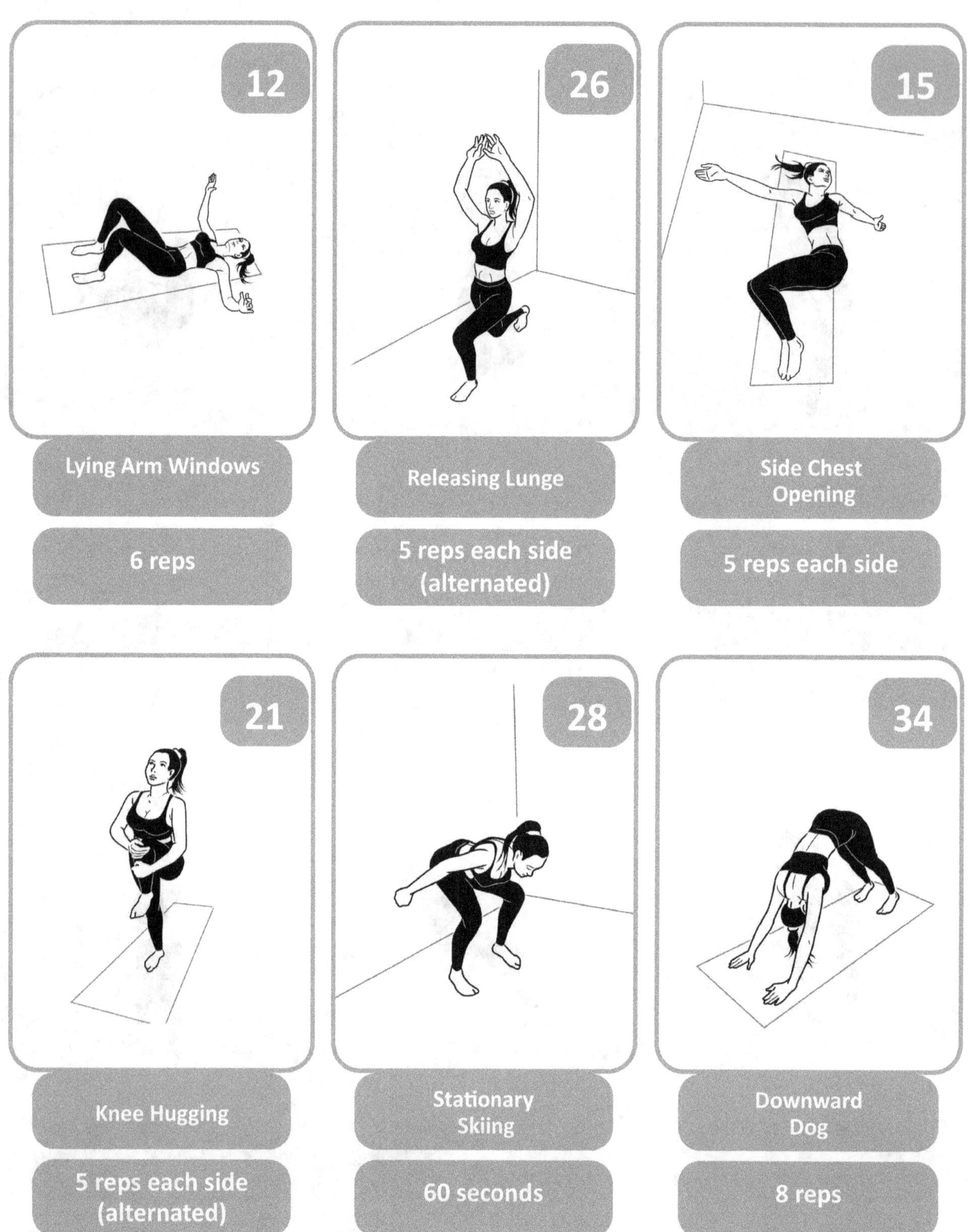

Day 17 - Repeat it three times.

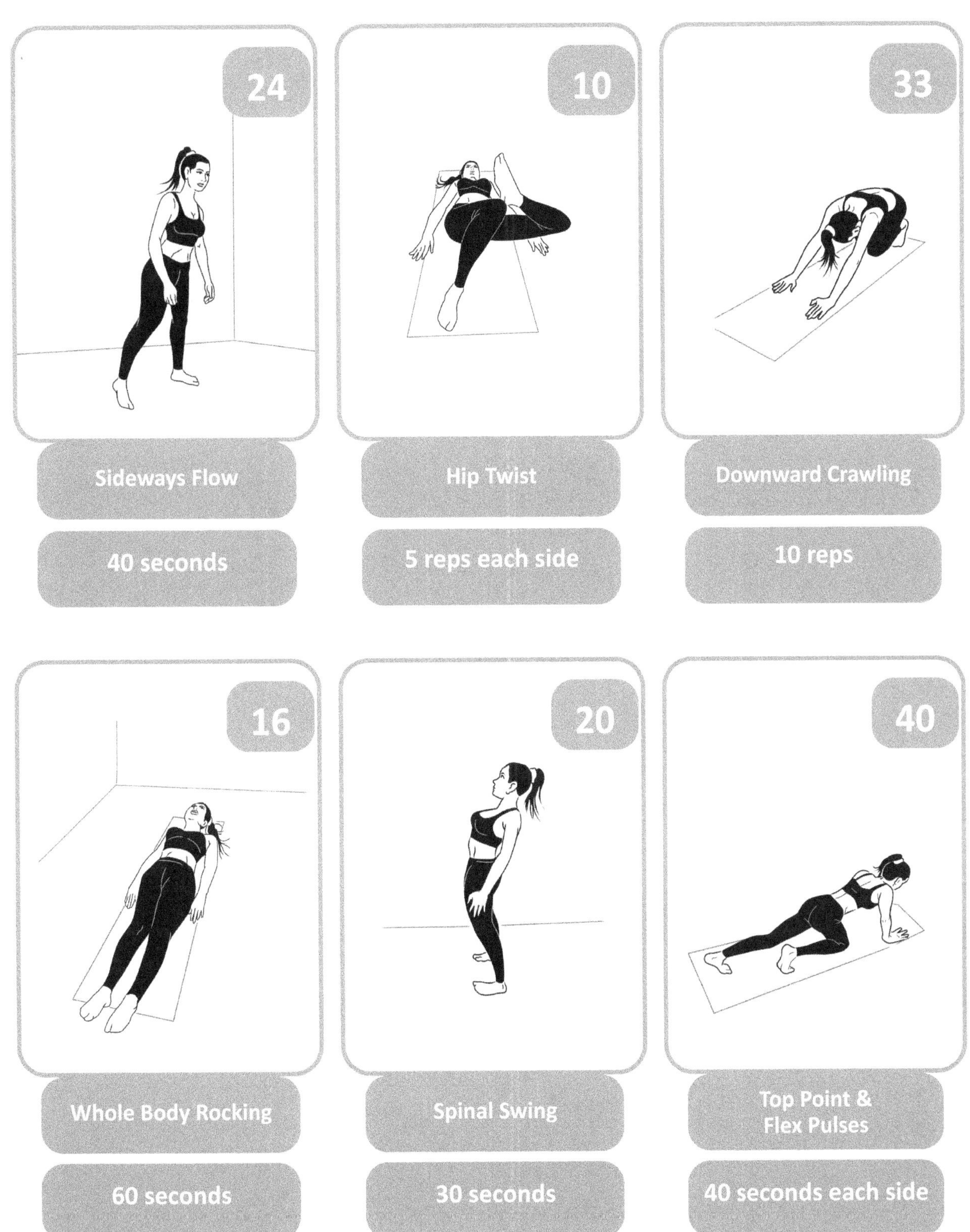

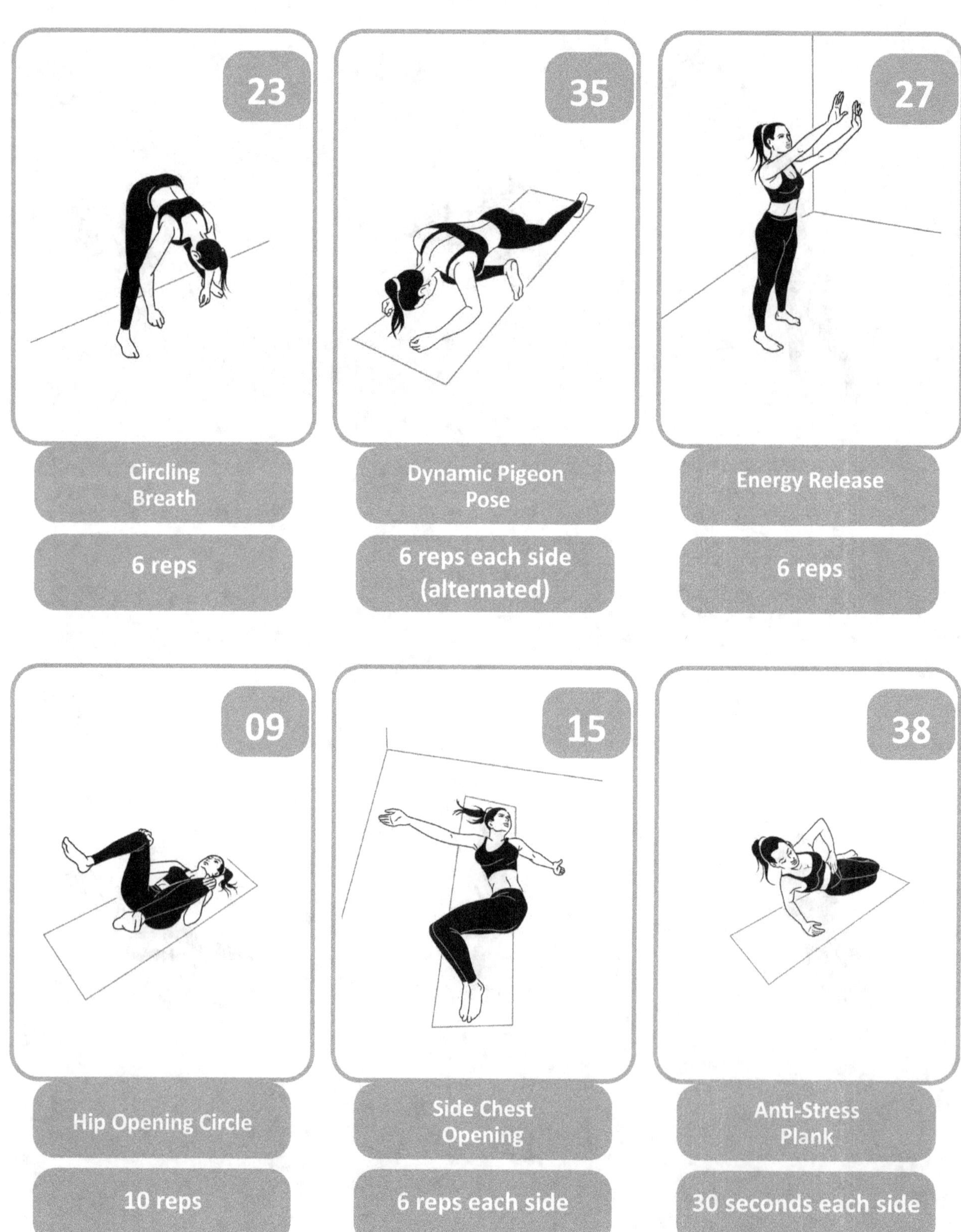
23
Circling
Breath
6 reps

35
Dynamic Pigeon
Pose
6 reps each side
(alternated)

27
Energy Release
6 reps

09
Hip Opening Circle
10 reps

15
Side Chest
Opening
6 reps each side

38
Anti-Stress
Plank
30 seconds each side

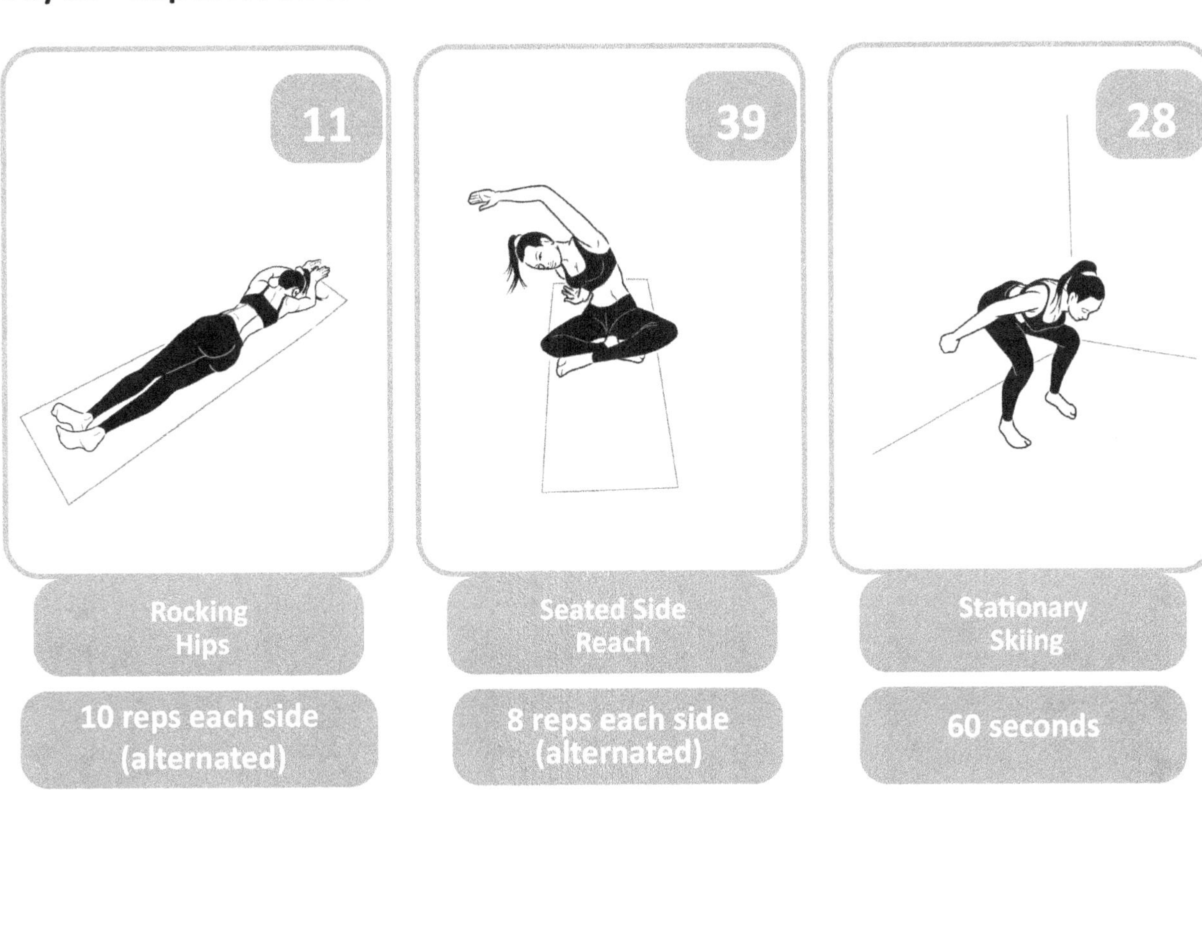

11	39	28
Rocking Hips	Seated Side Reach	Stationary Skiing
10 reps each side (alternated)	8 reps each side (alternated)	60 seconds

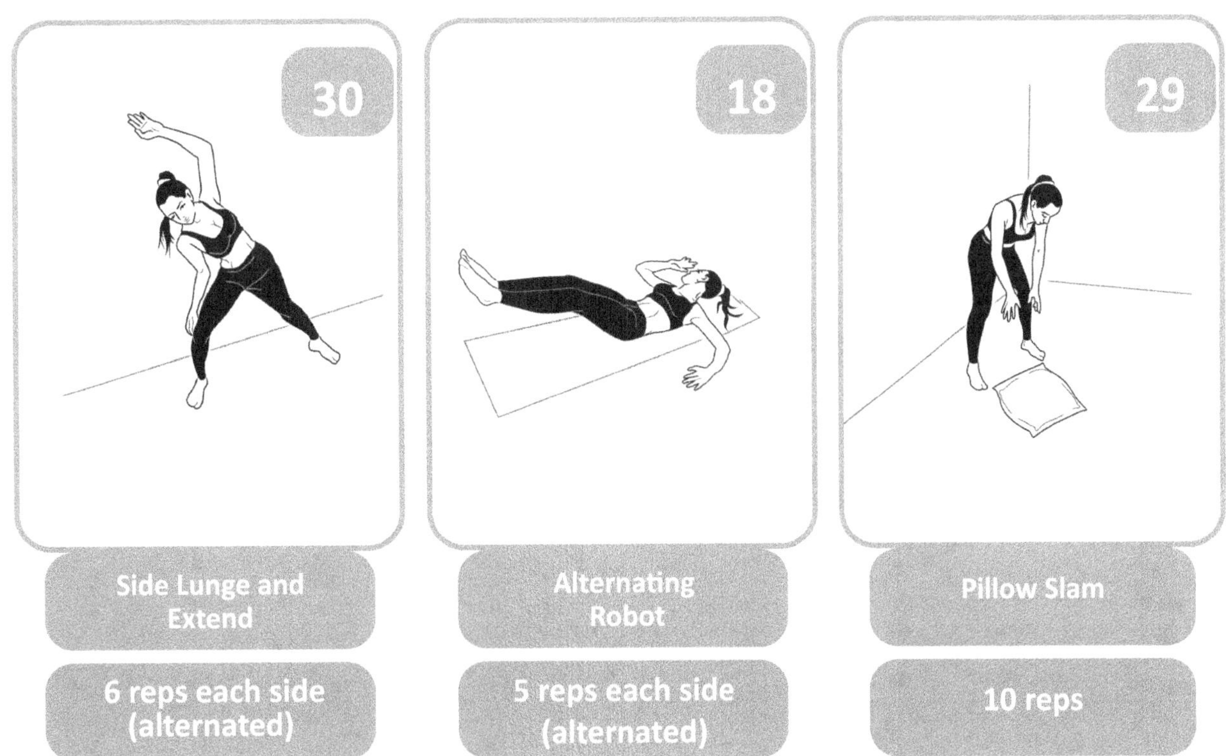

30	18	29
Side Lunge and Extend	Alternating Robot	Pillow Slam
6 reps each side (alternated)	5 reps each side (alternated)	10 reps

Day 20 - Repeat it three times.

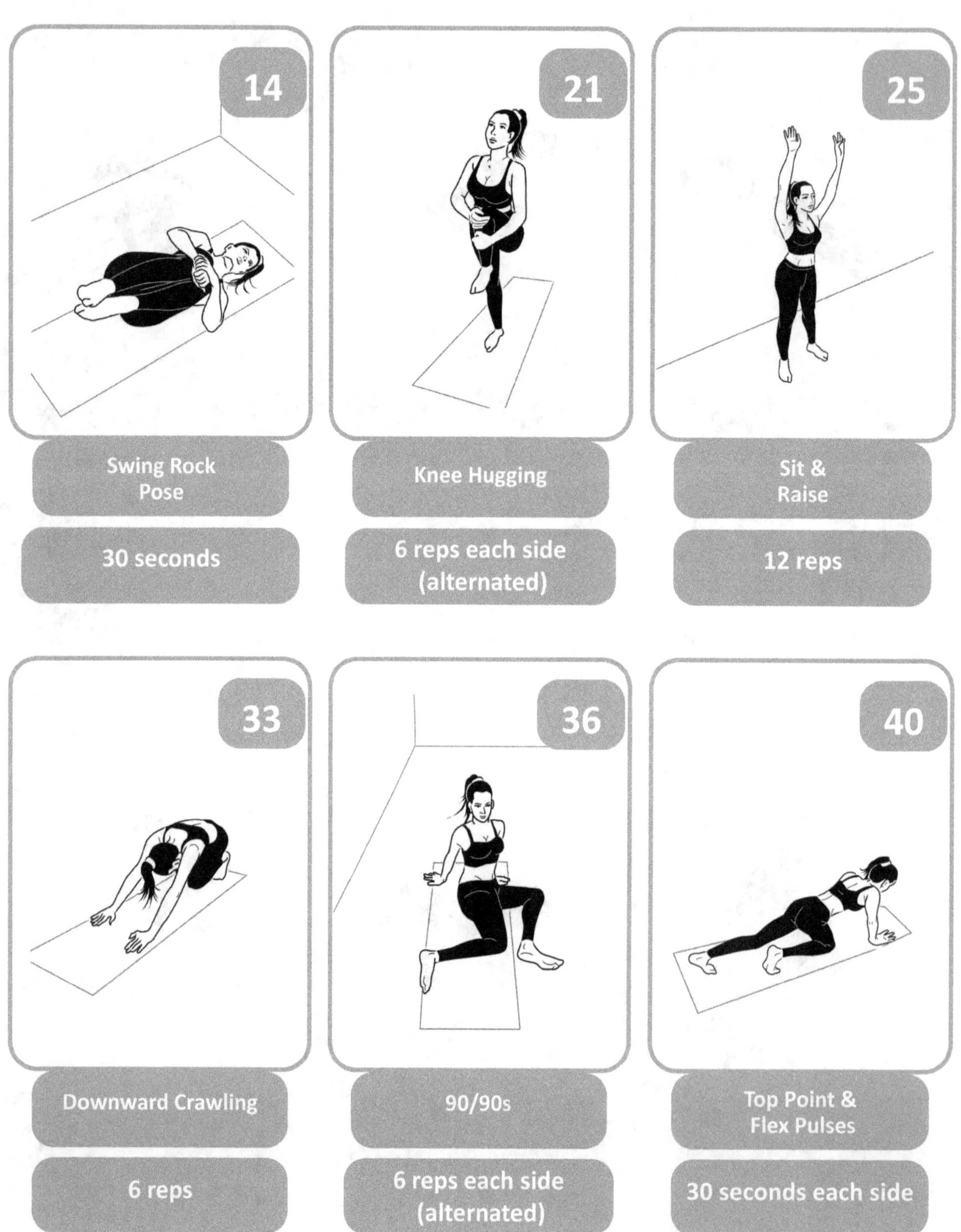

14	21	25
Swing Rock Pose	Knee Hugging	Sit & Raise
30 seconds	6 reps each side (alternated)	12 reps

33	36	40
Downward Crawling	90/90s	Top Point & Flex Pulses
6 reps	6 reps each side (alternated)	30 seconds each side

Day 21 - Repeat it three times.

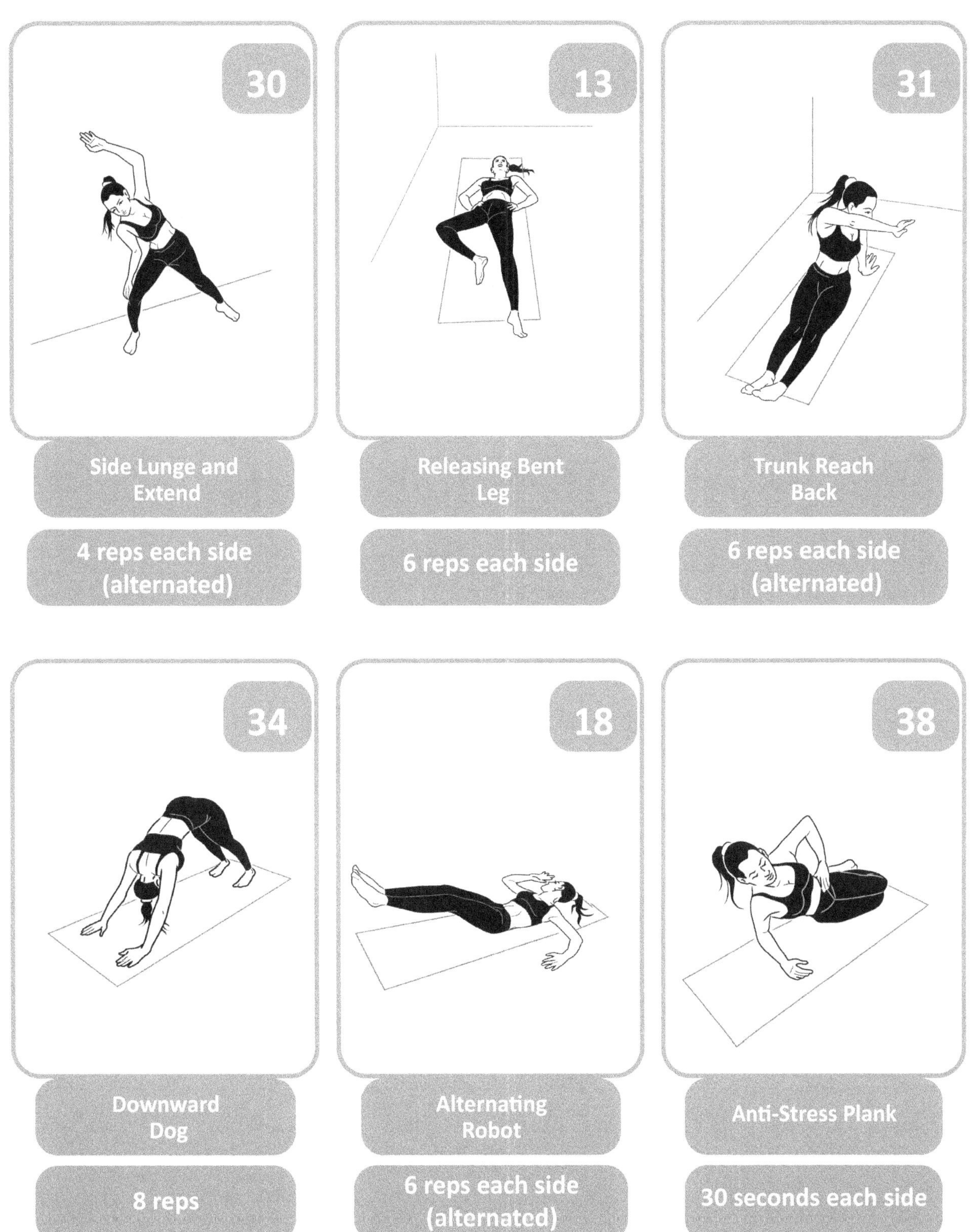

Day 22 - Repeat it three times.

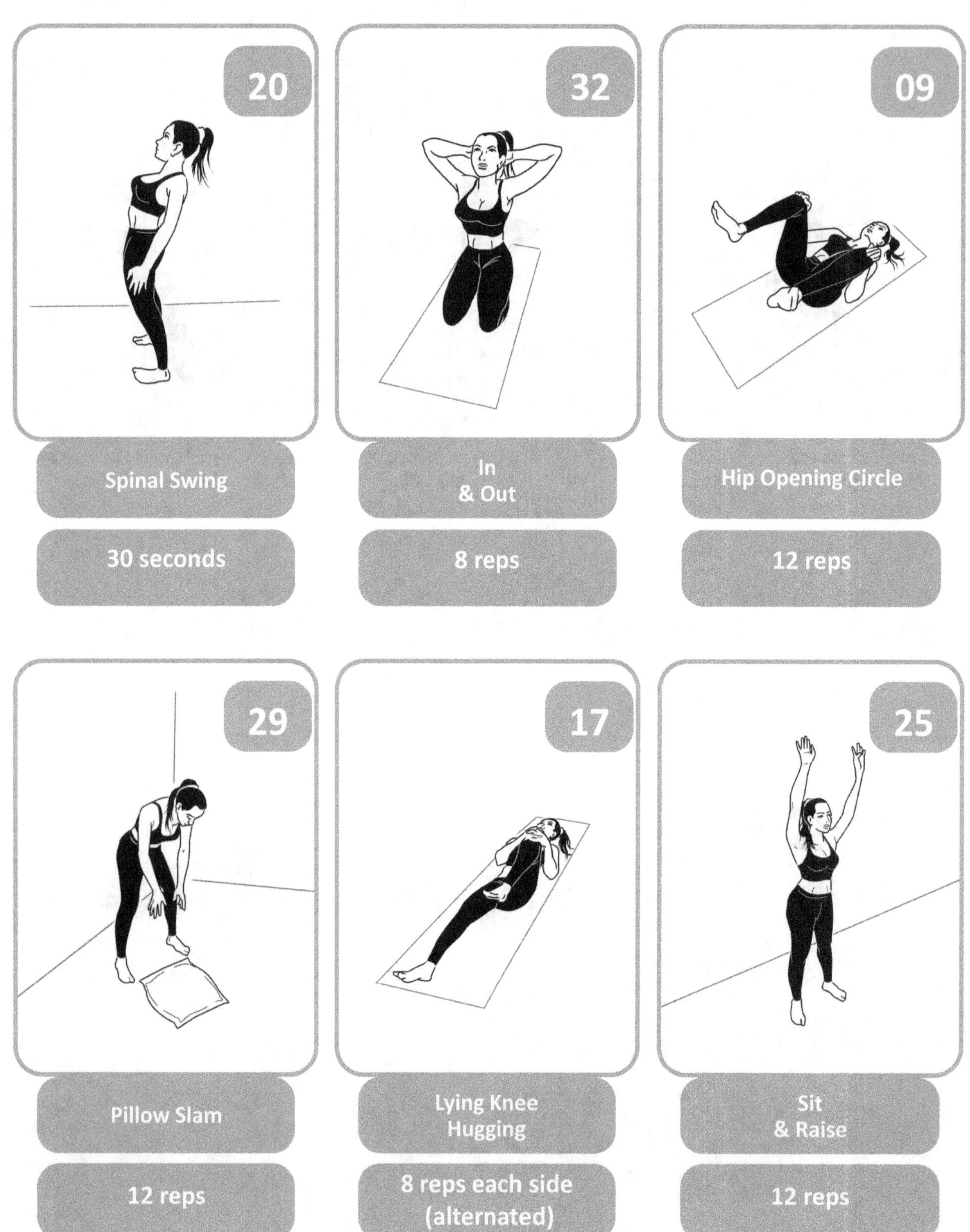

20 — Spinal Swing	32 — In & Out	09 — Hip Opening Circle
30 seconds	8 reps	12 reps
29 — Pillow Slam	17 — Lying Knee Hugging	25 — Sit & Raise
12 reps	8 reps each side (alternated)	12 reps

Day 23 - Repeat it four times.

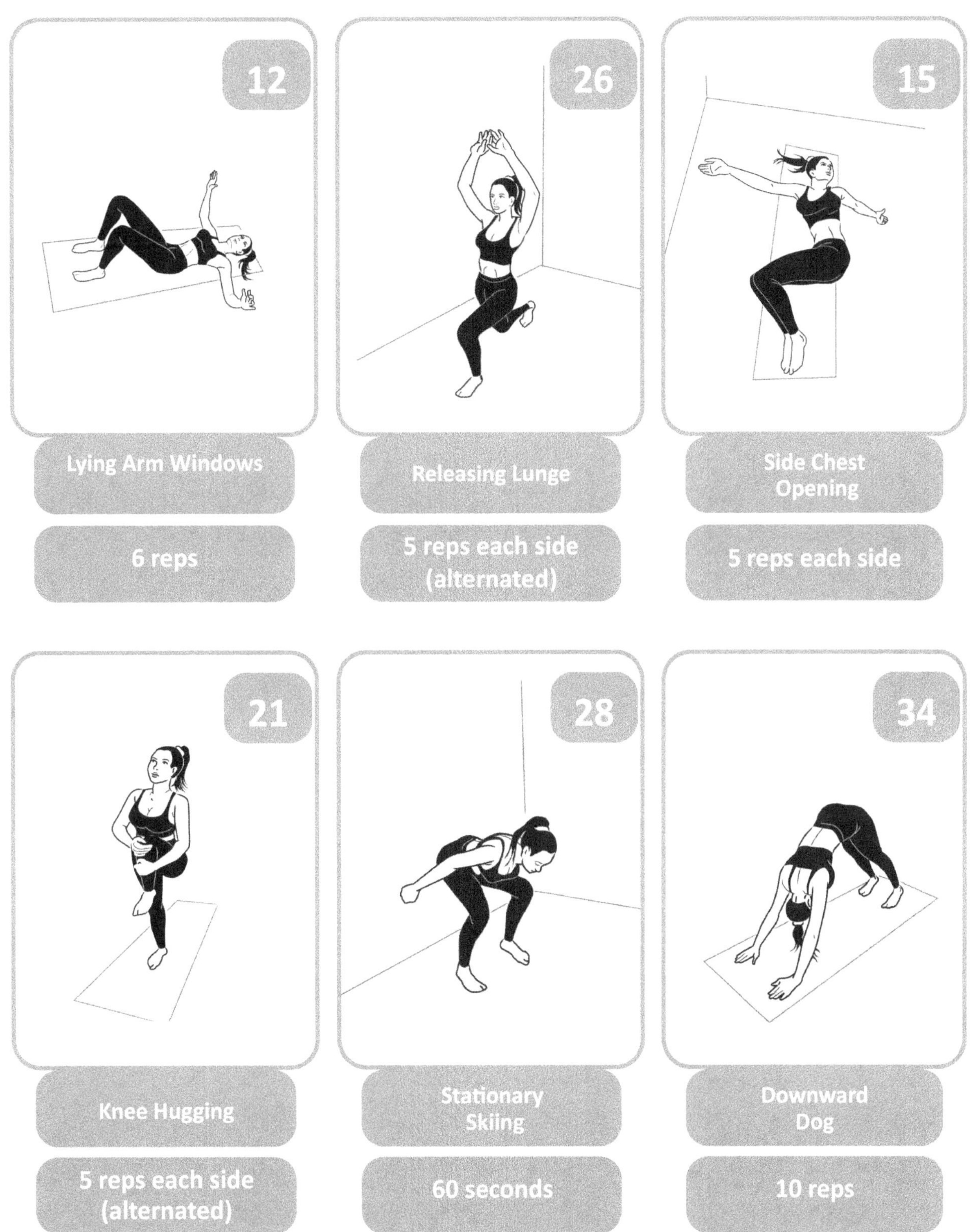

Day 24 - Repeat it three times.

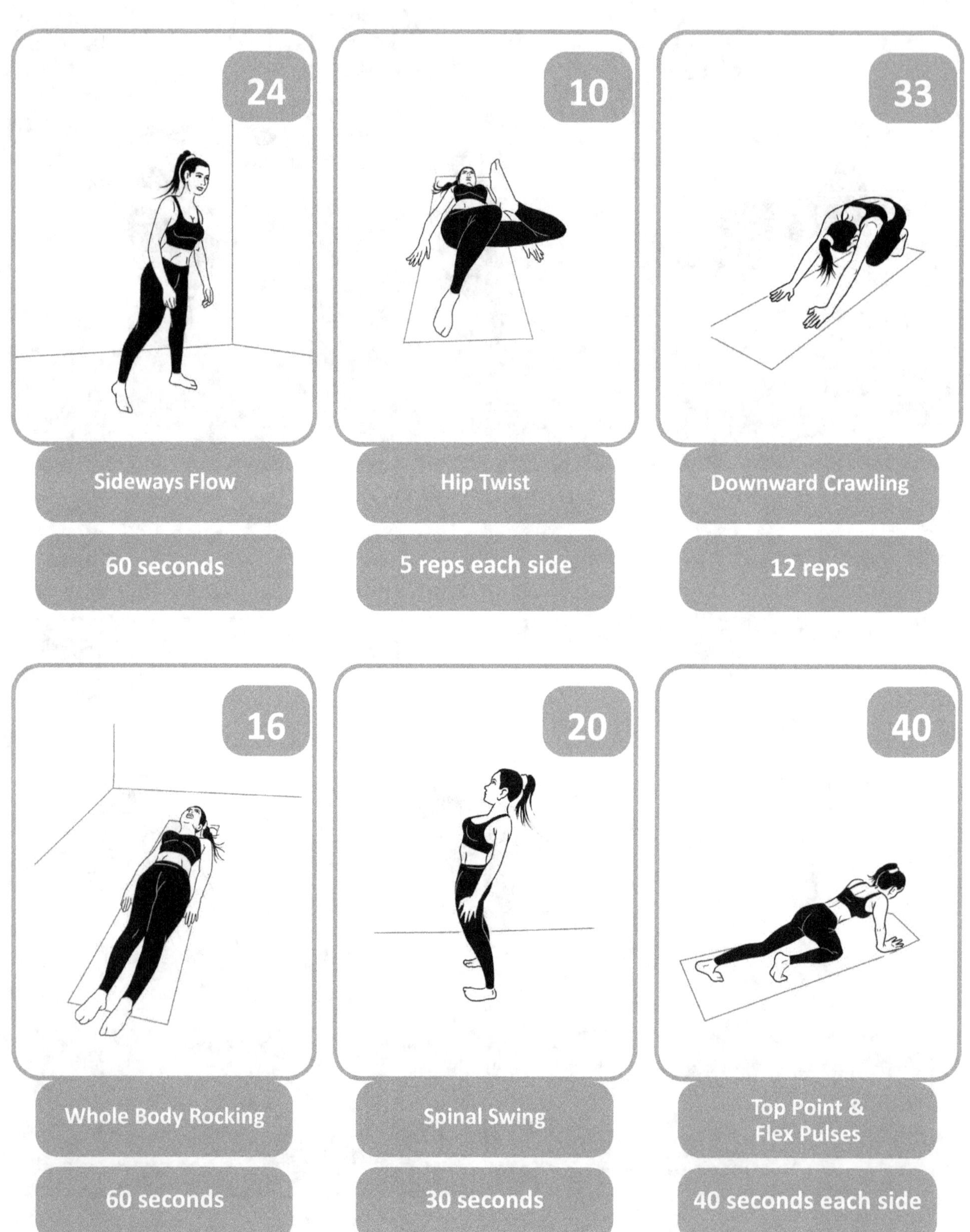

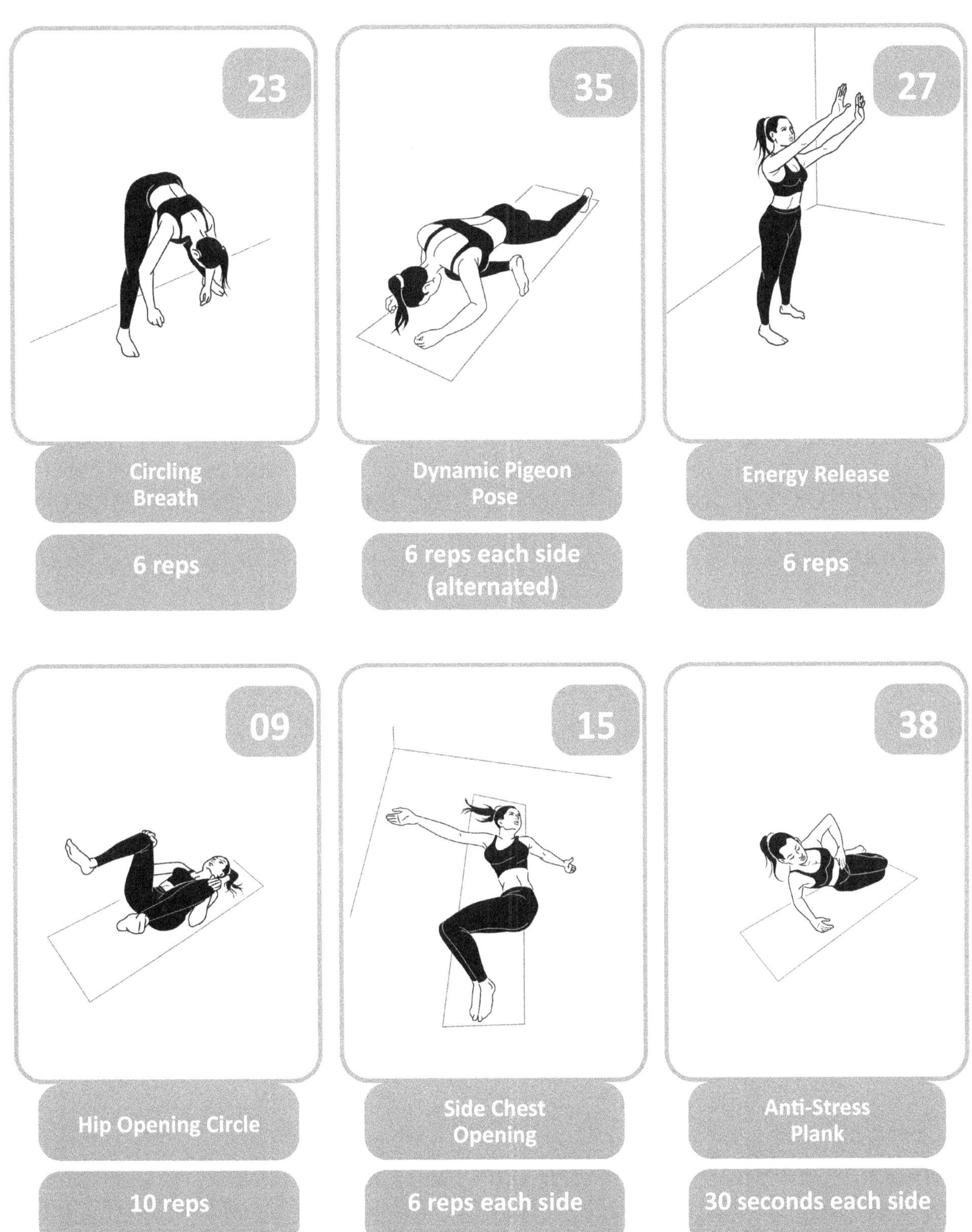

23
Circling
Breath
6 reps

35
Dynamic Pigeon
Pose
6 reps each side
(alternated)

27
Energy Release
6 reps

09
Hip Opening Circle
10 reps

15
Side Chest
Opening
6 reps each side

38
Anti-Stress
Plank
30 seconds each side

Day 26 - Repeat it three times.

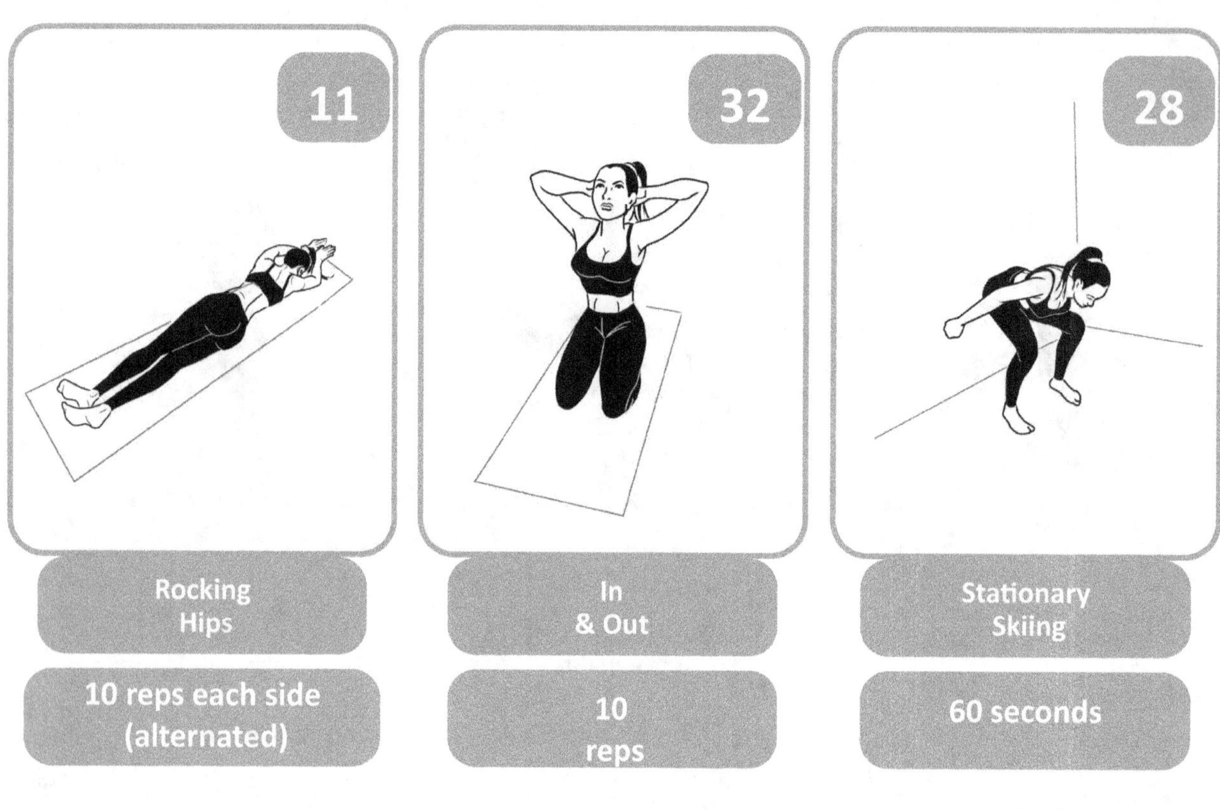

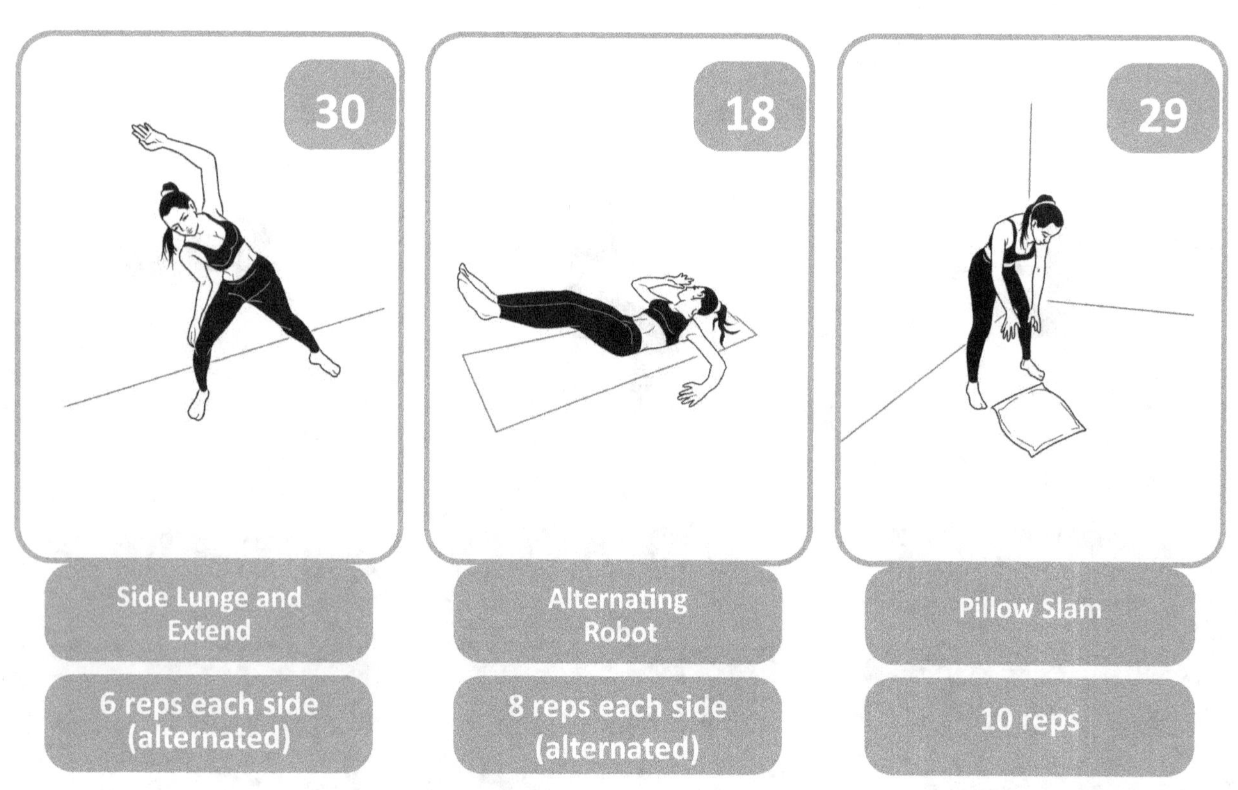

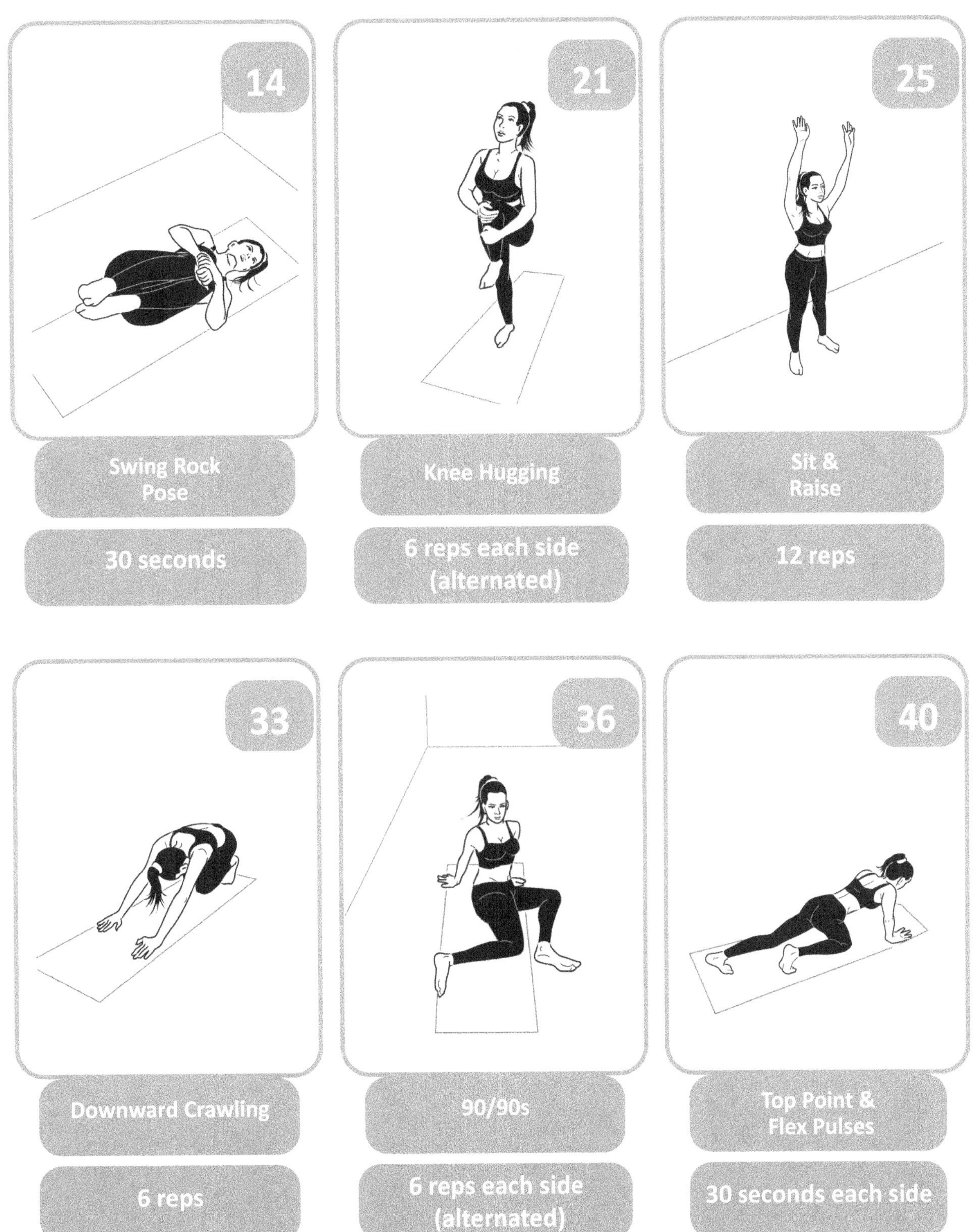

14
Swing Rock
Pose
30 seconds
21
Knee Hugging
6 reps each side
(alternated)
25
Sit &
Raise
12 reps
33
Downward Crawling
6 reps
36
90/90s
6 reps each side
(alternated)
40
Top Point &
Flex Pulses
30 seconds each side

Day 28 - Repeat it three times.

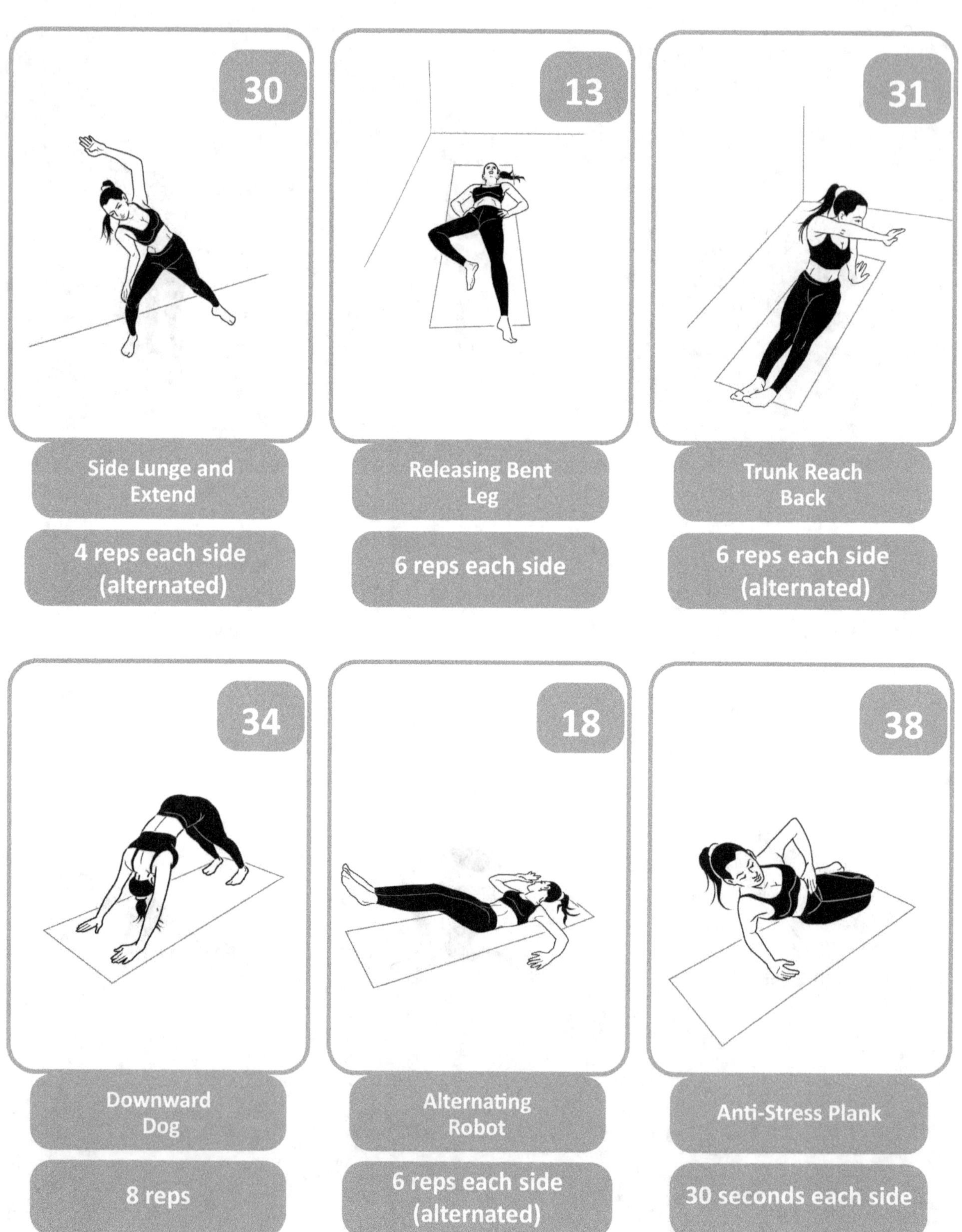

30	**13**	**31**
Side Lunge and Extend	Releasing Bent Leg	Trunk Reach Back
4 reps each side (alternated)	6 reps each side	6 reps each side (alternated)
34	**18**	**38**
Downward Dog	Alternating Robot	Anti-Stress Plank
8 reps	6 reps each side (alternated)	30 seconds each side

Well done for finishing those 28-days!

Now my recommendation is to take 3 days completely off from training (long walks are fine), and then restart from day 15 until 28, increasing one set for each workout (so instead of repeating the sequence three or four times, you go up to four/five times).

For any questions or doubts feel free to email me at
zealyonsfitness@gmail.com

CONCLUSION

Congratulations on finishing the book! I hope you enjoyed it! It is my sincere hope that it not only met, but exceeded your expectations, providing you with a new exercise repertoire and a better understanding of the transformative power of somatic practices.

I am confident that every one of the exercises included in these pages will help you open the door to a happier and healthier life. They are invaluable assets to both physical and mental health, as well as for releasing the stress and trauma that accumulates in life.

I send you my best wishes for happiness and success over the next few months. I hope this book helps you and serves as a reliable guide for you as you work towards better physical and mental health. I hope the exercises in this book give you joy and strength as you face life's challenges with courage and optimism.

If you have any questions or doubts, feel free to contact me at zealyonsfitness@gmail.com, and I'll be happy to assist you the best I can about somatic exercises and workouts!